A C
of Heart

A Change
of Heart

My Heart Transplant Journal
at the Freeman Hospital

Max Crompton

Jamble
House

Copyright © 2011 by Max Crompton

All rights reserved. No part of this publication may be
reproduced or transmitted in any form or by any means,
electronic or mechanical including photocopying, recording or any
information storage or retrieval system, without prior
permission in writing from the publisher.

The right of Max Crompton to be identified as the author of this
work has been asserted by him in accordance with the Copyright,
Designs and Patents Act 1988.

First published in the United Kingdom in 2011
by Jamble House

ISBN 978-0-9567955-0-2

Dedication

my donor – Andrew
my nephew – Jack
my best-friend's father – Steve
my fellow patient – Michael
sleep peacefully . . .

God Bless

"There is nothing more harmful to the soul, than an easy life"

T.Crompton

A Short Bit of Background

Hi. I'm Max. I don't know about you, but I can't stand reading introductions, or prefaces, or prologues, or whatever the hell these scholars want to call them. So I'll be as brief as possible, whilst still explaining enough for you to, hopefully, understand my Journal – my transplant story – better.

I am 27 years old and am the baby of my family; with an older brother, Tom and older still, twin sisters; Emma and Louise. I have been married for just under three years and me and my wife have a baby boy who is a mere 6 months old … and … I must say … bloody gorgeous!

In November 1982, 27 and a half years ago now, I was born with 'blue' lips and 'blue' fingertips. My local hospital took me away from my Mum and Dad straight away and rushed me to Great Ormond Street Children's Hospital (G.O.S.H), where I was diagnosed with Ebsteins anomaly – a malformation of the tricuspid valve, leading to poor function and enlargement of the right side of the heart.

When I was 14 I had open-heart surgery at G.O.S.H to repair the valve, then, two weeks later, the Surgeons went in again to replace the valve, as the repair was unsuccessful; I had a metal heart valve inserted that 'ticked' like a wrist watch – and as loud.

Other than those 6 weeks when I was 14 at G.O.S.H, I have led a relatively normal, good-quality life. I have always had a very low exercise capacity, which I will explain later, however, I have still led an active, happy life, enjoying many normal things throughout childhood and adulthood.

I had a scare with my heart in 2005, about a year after my father had passed away. At a routine check-up they saw that my heart had enlarged even further. I underwent several tests, however as there was no clinical change in me I was left alone to carry on as before.

Then, a year and a half ago, my heart become stuck in a fast heart rhythm. I was admitted to The Heart Hospital – the hospital you go to when you're too old for G.O.S.H – and was started on a medicine to slow my heart beat down.

24 hours after the medicine was given, I had a cardiac arrest – probably due to a rare side-effect of the medicine in conjunction with my heart condition. I was resuscitated and taken to Intensive Care (I.C.U), whereby I made a full recovery – the only difference being that I could no longer hear my metal valve 'tick'; peculiar, but I didn't think much of it, as I had made a full recovery.

However, 6 months later (one year ago now) at a routine outpatients check-up, they discovered that my metal valve was completely broken and was permanently fixed open. Also my heart on the right side was by now, so, so enlarged, it was barely beating at all. But what confounded the doctors the most was that I was still well; working, playing golf, walking – leading the same-old, good-quality life. But they knew that wouldn't last, because with my heart the way it was, all sorts of nasty, critical, fatal things could happen to me at any moment.

It was at this time that I was implanted with an I.C.D (an advanced pacemaker and defibrillator) to offer me some protection against a few of the dangers, but this was no long-term fix.

So although I was still showing no real symptoms of heart failure – I was still as well as I'd ever been – I was sent to The Freeman Hospital in Newcastle for a transplant assessment; The Freeman is the only Hospital in the UK that carries out transplants on patients with Congenital Heart Disease.

I was placed on the 'Active' transplant waiting list in November '09 (4 months ago), however, due to the nature of my extremely rare situation, I was admitted to The Freeman to wait, in their care, for a suitable donor.

So. My Journal starts on the day of admission on my journey to 'A Change of Heart'.

Journal One

WEEK 1 – ARRIVAL

30 March 2010 Tuesday

Wow. What a ride so far. Got the call from Newcastle on Thursday to tell me to move up today. Was a shock without being shocked, was a surprise which was unsurprising – was no more than the thundering rumble of inevitability. Yet it was and is, so scary.

I've often spoken of the two worlds that my life swings between. One healthy, happy and vivacious, the other dangerous, fatal and worrisome. One full of life, living and doing, the other void of safety, permanence, and peace. One fruitful, one fractious, one stable, one serious, one warm, one cold, one bearable, one not, one once present, but now passed – I'm now in the other world.

But let me tell you something and it's been true so far for all of my life, the worst of it all is not the other world – it's going from one to the other. It's leaving the light for the dark. That's the pain, and now I'm here, that awful, excruciating, chest-scything pain is now over. Phew!!! I am here. It is time. A world anew is calling.

I have a lovely room all to myself with a large window which faces east, so I can see the sunrise in the morning – my own bathroom and plenty of space. I'm tired because of the drive and the changing worlds, so early night I think – sleep please take me...

Day I in the Freeman house … 31/03/2010

Saw lots of people today. Transplant coordinators Lynne and Kirsty, head Surgeon Dr Asif Hasan, and a few other registrars and Amanda, the paediatric nurse.

Asif said that I will wait three months on average, however I scarcely believe he is being truthful with me although it may be true – I reckon he is being tactful to see what sort of person I am. Sounds bizarre but the world truly does work on our relationships with the people around us, despite contracts and protocols and due process – everything is people – and therefore everything at some point is subject to the subjectivity of the human soul – despite what systems there are or rules, if someone likes you, you will be so much better off.

That was pretty much it for the morning – Pam and Mum were having a nightmare trying to book viewings for renting a property. Bless Pam, she was getting so stressed and teary and kept apologising for drawing comfort from me, when the support should be going the other way, what with me being in hospital and being the one who has to go through the transplant – but she doesn't realise a few things: I said to her there is so much I want to do for her but can't because I'm in here. I said there's so many things I wish I could help her with but can't because I'm in here. I said there is so much I want to go and do with her but can't because I'm in here – so if giving her comfort and support and a shoulder to cry on is something that I actually CAN do, then I'll be damned if she thinks she can take that away from me through a mere misplaced sense of propriety and idealism.

I said to her let me have this, this small thing that I can do to help, let me comfort you and take any strength I can give you without comment or pause, because it's one of the only things, even being locked up in hospital, I can still do and I treasure it – so you can cry to me any time for your sake. She seemed to agree!! Yay!

Then better news came as Lynne came round and said that I was allowed outside and even out for a meal so don't think that I will be as limited as I first thought I might! Yay!! But very conscious of the fact that we have just got here and don't want to take any liberties too soon, so I'm still going to stay in the room most of the time to begin with.

Me, Mum and Pam went to Pizza Express at 6 PM though, which was lovely. We had two pizzas, two pastas and a side salad to share and us three ate every last morsel. We sat there eating, talking, drinking (I had a Coke – honestly) and had a real nice evening.

Can I actually really be on the heart transplant list? Is it really true??? I know the common X-Files phrase that 'the truth is stranger than fiction', but this reality really, really pushes the boundaries of natural intuition – but I suppose with hearts it's true that what you see (on the outside) is not what you get.

Got back to room and watched Arsenal versus Barcelona – Barcelona were so, so good. Maybe soon I can play football??? If it were I could fly. . .

Oh and forgot to mention Pam secured a rented house for £650 a month – three bedrooms, little garden, dining room and plenty of space all about ten minutes walk from the hospital, right next to the big lake and playing fields and park. It's perfect. I'm so pleased – only downside is that she can't move into it for another two weeks – but a small price to pay.

Day 2 – 01/04/10

Slept fretfully last night. Hospital beds are so uncomfortable when you are well. A thin, always over-starched, single sheet separating you from the plastic/rubber-mesh mattress. As soon as you get just a little bit too hot the merest hint of perspiration condenses on the barrier mattress and is absorbed by the paper thin sheet making it sodden and damp. So I move over a little to the other side of the mattress and start again. I suppose it isn't that bad – I mean the bed is soft and I have two pillows so I'm not too uncomfortable aside from my musing!

Found out today that my computer doesn't work here so Pam is going to drop it off to my work when she leaves tomorrow for them to fit it with a 3G dongle to whizz me up on the Internet. Then it should be all systems go! Bit of a pain because working here during work hours would be a real good pastime/time-killer, but hopefully I won't wait too long. Also work can only pay me in full if I'm actively working roughly full days so not too sure how long I can stay without my computer and still get paid. My work are really good so I don't think that will be a problem.

Had Echo today in my room by the special congenital heart technician with a seriously advanced echo machine. She was telling me of a two year old girl who had a heart transplant 10 days ago and is doing really well. It was done by Dr Hasan who I saw yesterday and it's just all so unbelievable – a two year old with an open chest and Dr Hasan taking out her heart. But the technician said relatively that heart transplants are the more simpler open-heart surgeries which is encouraging – Dr Hasan said that as well when we first met him.

10% chance of fatality. That's what my risk comes down to. Dr Hasan said previously that transplanting my heart will be straightforward, even with the Ebsteins and that because I'm so well and asymptomatic my chances of survival are 90% instead of the usual 80%.

But how hard is it to assimilate numerical percentages with instinctual fear? How absurd is it a task to temper emotive responses with logical statistics? I wonder, at the point when I'm laying on the surgical bed and I have the Anaesthetists buzzing around me, and I have an oxygen mask on and they are saying I'll start to feel drowsy and drift off, I wonder, in that moment, will I be scared? And if I am, will the statistical knowledge matter at all?

In those last waking moments, will I be as scared of them being my last waking moments ever, if it were 95%? 97%? 82%? 76%? 70%? 98%? 60%? Any percent? I get the feeling that those last moments on the trolley before I go under will be the same no matter what number is written on the consent form under risks. I will still, I reckon, feel the same – whatever it is I will be feeling. Fear, I fear, is unassuaged by logic.

Man that will be scary though won't it – when the 'time' finally arrives. But I sometimes forget that we have already been through the process of actually having the Op. Okay it was called off before I was on the operating trolley but it wasn't much before that...

*   *   *

In December, on a Friday evening, when we were at home, we were called up for the transplant. Half hour after Newcastle called us that night an Ambulance picked me and Pam up and rushed us straight onto the main runway at Stansted Airport, whereby we were flown by private jet to Newcastle. It was just crazy. The transplant didn't happen in the end, because upon retrieval the donor's heart was enlarged and had something wrong with the ventricle walls too, so it was a no-go.

But I've never felt anything like it. I've never experienced a stronger or more powerful tirade of emotions. I'd even say the feeling goes deeper than feelings themselves.

It's like on the surface and facing the world is your ego and normal personality – then just under your surface, in the shallows, there's your inner feelings and reacting emotions – then down in the depths, at the bottom of the deepest ocean ridge is your inner self – all ways laid bare, all feelings and thoughts at their most elemental state – what could be seen as the cornerstone of everything you are.

It is this unfettered and untainted place I've been before with my heart problems – when Dad was taken from us – with Pam being ill – and with Pam's love and the birth of Alex. Some people, like Tom, would say how privileged I have been to have gone to this place so many times – and when I ponder it I probably agree with him.

However, that night I got the call for the transplant with total shock and surprise, I found, it seems now, another depth, another inner layer of myself – a state almost intranscendental to the world even at the base of the deep ocean ridge. This is what I mean by what I felt wasn't even a 'feeling', it was deeper than that.

The moment specifically was when me and Pam were in Alex's room – he was peacefully asleep, soaring the highest clouds in his dreams no doubt – and I kissed him and said 'goodbye.'

This moment exactly was when I'd experienced what I've just pathetically tried to describe. My legs almost buckled under me in that room after I leaned over and kissed his Alex-scented cheek – but I didn't know I had legs at the time. I was crying – apparently – I couldn't feel my tears. I was close to hyperventilating – I wasn't aware I even needed to breathe.

I have never known anything close to that before – never. I have thought about it lots since and tried to understand it – what with Alex being my son who, at 3 months old, doesn't yet know me and wouldn't yet remember me. I suppose it's this fact, sunk in the sea of Love I have for him, that tore me down to less than even my base parts.

I was okay with myself, and Pam and Mum when the call came – terrified and feeling a million things, most of all overwhelming love – however it was Alex, the addition of my only baby son caught up amongst all this that took me to that strange, strange place.

I can't even use fear or love or hope to describe that place because this seemed to come before them. I suppose it is as close to this 'other state' that Plato and Blake and Zen refer to that I'll ever get. Man that night was crazy – everything turned into one and life and everything dissolved into an indescribable thing;

> *'To see a world in a grain of sand*
> *or Heaven in a wildflower*
> *to hold Infinity in your hand*
> *and eternity within an hour'*

I don't think it will be quite like that again to be honest – well I suppose I'm hoping it won't be!!

*   *   *

Anyway the Echo was the only medical happening of the day. There was much hot debate as to the arrangements for moving Alex, Pam's Dad and all our stuff up here, however we eventually decided.

The problem was that the house doesn't become available until two weeks yesterday – but Pam had booked her ticket home Friday to get back to Alex. Mum was going back home Monday and everyone – Pam, Alex, John, Mum, Louise and all our stuff were going to come back up Thursday week! Although we could move in (don't know why I'm saying 'we'), on Wednesday (the 14th), Pam's brothers Kev and Pete, who are driving Pam and Alex and John and all our belongings up cannot do it on the Wednesday. But the big problem with all of this is that I would be left on my own for nine whole days and Pam would be away from me for a whole two weeks.

At first I said that would be all right because I knew Pam had to get back to Alex and I didn't want her doing too much (she has only recently made a full recovery from Toxic Shock). However, as the day went on Pam, who never liked the plan, become even more agitated with it.

In her words she knows Alex is extremely well looked after by her Dad and sister Jen, and that out of the two of us, Alex and me, her time is more needed in the company of me. She said if Alex was in hospital then it would be the other way round. It's whoever needs her the most, that's where Pam wants to be – and at the moment, Pam says, that need is with me – don't tell anyone but I'm so glad she thinks that!

So we changed the plans slightly so she would go home tomorrow as planned, but then come back the Friday after. Therefore I'll only be on my own for three days – Tuesday, Wednesday and Thursday, so will be much better for us all – most of all me!!

So, John and Jen will have Alex Friday to Thursday (15th) then Mum and Louise will fly up with Alex; John will come up with all our stuff driven by Pam's brother Kev – so sorted!!

Went for a lovely meal at Mum' s Hotel – The Jesmond. Three fine, unbelievably nice courses for £13.95 only. I have never ever seen such good value for money – if you saw and tasted the food you'll know what I mean.

But it was then the last night with Pam for a whole week and when we got back to the hospital Pam was really upset. Probably the most upset I've seen her in a long time. We were standing, freezing, cuddling, outside the hospital before we both went our separate ways – me to Ward 30, Pam to the hospital residential flat Beachwood.

She was really sobbing telling me how much she loves me and how that being with me has been the happiest time of her life. She kept saying you're everything to me Max, you're everything. Was heart-wrenching to hear – the love she has for me is remarkable, as I her.

I was squeezing her so tight my arms ached. The cold weather, the wind, the chill of the northern air could no longer penetrate us ... In that moment we were warm in each other's arms, we were both safe in each other's arms, we were one, in no longer the others' arms.

I just scrunched and scrunched and scrunched her, telling her it would be okay. You see when Pam goes back home it will be quite possible that if I did get called for the transplant, she would not be able to get back up to me in time before I get taken off to theatre – so I think that was on her mind a lot.

I just comforted her and reminded her that this was not goodbye! Bless her. I could use up all the air in this world telling you about the wonder and glory of Pam and I wouldn't even be half done. I could use all known languages, past and present, to tell you how much that girl does for me, but they would barely get me started. I could reuse all the ink that has ever been written to tell you how much Pam means to me, but it would not suffice, not even close, nowhere near.

As I was comforting her she kept telling me how strong I was to yet again be comforting her and that she was the weak one. Tut-tut-tut dear child, I should have said – you think that's my strength that I'm radiating? You think the resolve and level-headedness and grace that you see in me at the moment is all mine? Well it's not. No way.

I should have said to her if you want to know my secret, if you want to know how I can be so strong, and face perils with smiles and hope, and comfort you and stay sane and keep going, keep, keep going no matter what, then you should go back to your room – over to the dresser and look into the mirror – that's where you'll find the answer.

As we were huddled outside the hospital I heard someone call out 'Max'. We looked up and saw the couple we flew back with the night I was called up for my transplant (in December). Can't remember their names – although they could mine which speaks highly of them – but they are a, say, 40 year old husband and wife from Belfast – the wife was needing a double lung transplant.

She had her transplant two weeks ago and she was looking so very well. She was in a wheelchair still, but didn't have any tubes, or drips and most importantly wasn't on any oxygen – which she had been on constantly for about two years I think.

They were just moving into the hospital flats and it looked like it was all going so well for them. They were flown over four times for transplantation, but each time it was called off at the last minute, so they are so pleased now. She just looks so well and so soon after transplant, it's just amazing!

Then went back to my room to bed – with a well full tummy!

Day 3 – 02/04/10

Pam visited early but had to leave at 8:15 AM for the train so that was a bit of a bummer.

Me and Mum then read my book 'To Kill A Mockingbird' a little and played cribbage in the canteen which was really funny. To be fair to Mum she picked it up really well, but she was still doing some crazy things. Whilst pegging she opened with a 10 and said two points?? And she had this fascination about 7s, that they meant something special?

To be fair I am no Oracle on cribbage and her dad played it a lot apparently so there maybe something about 7s I don't know about – however, this is coming from someone who deliberately left her passport and photo-card driver license at home with the intention of flying back from Newcastle to London on no more ID than her bank debit cards and BACP counselling membership card!! Hah-hah, but I suppose it is only an internal flight, so thinking you don't need your passport isn't so bad, but no photo ID is pushing it a bit too far I think.

As ever Mum has been so, so wonderful. Always there, patient, easy-going, unobtrusive and such a good stress reliever. She really is a remarkable woman, a mother to the core who sets an example for all of us.

She is the other woman in my life who I'd be lost without. I know they say behind every good man there is a good woman, but in my case I think, behind me there are two great women.

That evening I had my first real 'wobble'. Just before Mum left at around 6 PM I got my funny vision thing on my right side (a panoramic arc of wishywashyness forms on my right side of vision) – like a crescent moon of water toward the right edge of wherever I look.

Get it every now and again when I am really tired, or knackered, or run down. Usually doesn't last long and have had it since I was a teenager – apparently others get it too so it really is nothing at all to worry about, but it was enough to make me feel edgy!

Mum had just left and the room, which was turning to twilight because of the tinted windows and Pam was hundreds of miles away and I just had that horrible, uneasy, lost, lonely type of feeling roll all over me. And my vision was making it all seem scarier.

So went for a walk in the brisk air and walked around the whole hospital which took about 15-20 minutes – it's a really large hospital. Cleared up my vision completely, really quickly – the cold air always does, so when I got back I felt okay really – but realised one resounding fact – absolutely no way can I be left on my own in Newcastle, whilst everyone else is down south.

Although I may have been okay being away from everyone as things are, the thought that I could really, really, really, at any moment, be taken to transplant, means there's no way I could do that by myself. No way. In my first little wobble I realised that completely and thought how stupid I had been to think that I could last three days – or, hell, the 11 days we first thought by myself. It was just madness – utter madness!

It's all okay when everything is okay for Pam and Mum to be miles away, but the second I have another 'wobble', or actual transplant call, then I would crumble to bits – or at least go to. Why make it harder on myself than it already is, aye?

So change of plan – Mum will go home Tuesday, and Pam will come back up then too. Then the Thursday week later Kev will drive John and all our stuff up and Mum and Louise will fly up with Alex. Sorted.

This is only possible because John and Jen will look after Alex solely again for another nine days – it's just such a godsend having a father and sister in-law like those two. The amount they do for us and care for me makes me sort of want to omit the 'in-law' when referencing their relation to me. I cherish them way more than they know. They have done so much and helped beyond measure.

Was my worst night yet that night though. I just couldn't get to sleep and really don't want to get into the habit of asking for sleeping tablets, especially not so early on. I could be here months and if I start asking for sleeping tablets now, by the time I get home I'd have forgotten the natural process of drifting off to sleep permanently – okay maybe a bit of an over exaggeration!!

Anyway, tossed and turned until 1 A.M. and could not get asleep. There was a TV blaring the whole time and I was getting more and more worked up by it. At 1:30 AM I buzzed the nurse to ask to see if they could turn it down – she knocked on the door next to me (this Scouser) and he said no worries – or something like that. Couldn't really hear but he sounded nice. But the noise didn't go away. Just a blaring TV.

At 2 AM now I thought 'sod it' and got up to investigate myself. Guess what? The TV was blaring from a cubicle which was empty!! All that time tossing and turning and putting my head under the pillow and putting my Alice band over my ears and the TV was left on in an empty room. Arghhhhhh!!!! I shut it off and went back to bed.

Then had a real, real good cry. Stuffed my face deep into my pillow to mute the noise. My pillow was wet when I stopped. I was crying for the sole reason of intimate loneliness. In short, I so miss cuddling up to Pam's gloriously warm gorgeous body – and together floating away to a gentle sleep . . . it will be a while until we can do that again – but I'll take that so long as it does happen again. . . . I know it sounds depressing, but total positivity is nothing more than delusion. Although I accept that many people may disagree. I fell asleep eventually – say a bit after 2 AM.

Day 4 – 03/04/10

Had quite a nice day today. Talked and played more cribbage with Mum as you can see with the scores [*original journal contained cribbage scoring table*]. The last game to the left she was on fire – scoring points at will and finished perfectly in the hole from 15 points out – amazing. Blind luck of course!! Only jesting.

Dr Hasan came around in the morning again with consultant Dr Choudhury. Am surprised how much of the surgeon I've seen, but think he is more of a consultant figure as well as the lead surgeon. He does have such a presence about him. A sort of magisterial, presidential aura about him which is shown as much by the way the other doctors and staff are around him, than by him in himself. He conveys a feeling of utter competence and care and, I suppose, control. He is someone that I reckon always has the floor wherever he goes and everyone always stops talking as he walks in and everyone would always stand slightly behind him when entering a room. But he is very nice and seems to have 'time' for you which the high-up medical consultants/surgeons do not usually give you – so shows how much he does and how thorough, I suppose, he is.

I mean I've seen him three separate times since I've been here already which is more than you would ordinarily expect for my whole stay. But the staff do say how committed he is and just how much he does for his patients.

Apparently, according to the paediatric nurse Amanda, he is probably the best congenital heart surgeon in the country, and one of the main reasons that the 'Institute of Transplantation', a national centre for transplantation – the first of it's kind, is currently under construction here at the Freeman and not in London or elsewhere more central. I suppose that can only fill you with confidence can't it?

Just after 5 PM me and Mum walked over to where Pam is going to be living and we saw what looked like an Italian restaurant. As we got closer to it though we saw it was an Italian delicatessen cafe. Lots of really nice looking pastas and pizzas and really good quality Italian food. Also it is a deli so real nice looking balsamic vinegars and white bean and Pomodoro preserves and pickles and pastas and Moretti and all sorts that you can buy.

Considering how much me and Pam love Italian-food then this cafe/deli is just a perfect thing to have opposite. However, as we got there it was just closing so we couldn't have dinner there that night. And because it's Easter they won't be open again until Tuesday, still, it's not like I'm in a rush now is it?

So we headed back and I had dinner in my room. Was raining whilst we were out and got quite heavy so I looked like a drowned rat once I got back to the ward. There I was, drenched, in my Merrill trainers, Superdry jogging bottoms, jumper and coat and I could not have looked further from a hospital inpatient – more like an ill-prepared hiker. I looked so out of place going back to my room and I haven't got a hospital wristband yet, so I really do look like an out of hours visitor!!

Food that night was well nice – mulligatawny soup and sweet and sour pork and rice. So nice. I honestly can't believe how nice the hospital food is here! It is always piping, piping hot, really tasty and even the veg is not steam cold mush, but warm and slightly crunchy. It will be absolutely no hardship at all eating exclusively hospital food for a while.

Oh, I tell you that night I had a real newby to my obs (observations – blood pressure/ SATs /pulse/temperature). You always do encounter nurses like him. Really nice, new, polite, and dreadfully over-keen. I think the more experience you get the more common sense you gain and therefore do not need to follow the 'house nurse operating rules' book to the very letter.

First he asks me if I'm in any pain, which isn't so bad as it's a standard question to ask, even though the more adept nurses can see they don't need to ask it. Then he does my temperature – he jabs the ear thermometer more into the side of my ear than into the channel – oh no I've right got one here!! Then he does my blood pressure, pulse and SATs without a hitch, so I thought maybe I'd judged him too soon, but wait for it… he took the Velcro pad off and I went to lay back down – expecting him to disappear out the room when he said he also had to measure my respiratory rate – I tell you no nurse has ever measured my respiratory rate!

So he stood there, watching me breathe, counting my breaths – looking at my chest for 30 seconds. Super, super keen. I reckon it was his first day on work experience bless him.

Then he asked if I wanted my bed raised – 'no' I assured him. Then he said do you want the foot rest thing at the end of the bed pulled out further – 'no thanks' I said. Then he said is there anything else that I wanted…… 'Get lost. I'm trying to get asleep. It's 10:30 PM and you've turned my light on' I wanted to say – but of course I just said 'no thanks, thanks very much'.

I don't intend to sound arrogant, even though I probably do. He was really, really nice and I suppose he has to do all that, but, boy, when you're trying to get asleep, the last person you want to come in to do your obs is a super over-keen nurse.

Oh no………. he is on again tonight!!!

Day 5 – 04/04/10 (Easter Sunday)

Easter Sunday is like Christmas day in terms of bank holidays – nearly every shop is shut, no newspapers are printed – and nothing at all happens at hospital. Didn't see anyone today and the corridors and car parks and the usual buzz of the hospital is, today, empty, lethargic and subdued. So had a real slow uneventful day – played cribbage with Mum, she still can't fully get the pegging points around the 31 for 2 points, or 31 for 3 points if it's the last card!

Am so enjoying spending all this time with Mum. She makes hour's float so easily by – will be sad to see her go Tuesday. We went to her digs at Beechwood for a little and the canteen, but the real good part of the day was when we went walking, directly opposite the hospital, into Paddy Freeman's Park and the river valley beyond.

I can't believe how beautiful it is. Directly opposite the hospital is a stretching park, beyond which is a small river. However, the Paddy Freeman Park is on high ground, so once you cross through it you're met with this deep ravine which cuts downward – steep and fast – to the river below.

The river is more of a stream – it's small and windy. So when you look out you feel like you're atop a cliff with a deep view of the territory below – which is a labyrinth of tall old trees, inter-twined and interlocked all the way down to the stream where there is a fast flowing waterfall. Once you get to the edge and look down you're met with this wonderful winter forest vista with the pounding of rushing water echoing strongly up the valley.

There are footpaths and old stone bridges all along the stream and down through the valley – we saw lots of hikers out with their maps trundling the valley floor – it must be a good few hundred feet from the top of the Park down to the riverbed below. It's like stepping out of the hospital, crossing the road and within a matter of a couple of dozen steps you're immersed

in nature like on a walking holiday. Also there is a lovely kids'
play area and big lake with ducks so Pam, Alex and John will just
love it here. I tell you other than family and friends and our
lovely house we would probably not want to go home it's so
lovely up here.

Bought a 12 day TV pass for £20 today – so expensive – and
watched Jonathan Creek Easter special. Was actually quite
rubbish for Jonathan Creek's standards. Then F.W.A.F (Four
Weddings and A Funeral) was on – so funny;

Film Quotes

'Bride or groom?'
'Pardon?'
'Bride or groom?'
'I should think it's quite obvious I am neither...'

'Hi I'm Charles'
'Don't be ridiculous Charles died five years ago'
'I think perhaps another Charles?'
'Are you trying to tell me I don't know my own brother?'

So funny. Took ages to get to sleep again and I was cold as well
which didn't help. But once I drifted off it was okay. Had
horrible nightmare though – can't really remember what about
but I groaned and actually woke myself up!! Handy aye?

WEEK **2**

Day 6 – 05/04/10

Woke up still cold. Weather looks like a depressing grey mush and it's raining. Looking out of the window it could not be more drab, miserable and depressing; grey soup pouring with rain – everywhere there is just land then grey – no further definition at all. Nice. No walking today me thinks. And I'm Still Cold! I'm never cold – where's my jumper? Oh here it is. Oh but I know I've got to have a shower. Shucks! I well can't be arsed. Boredom breeds lethargy I feel – and from there it's just a short hop-skip-and-jump to indifference. And that would turn into depression before you could say 'fed up'. I must stay active – I must stay focused – I must refuse to be discouraged!

Started getting quite a few arrhythmias for some reason for an hour or two. Had a couple of bananas and some water and played some more cribbage to take mind off it and it soon went.

Spent up to lunchtime in the room just in case anyone came round, but didn't see anyone.

Mum's writing;

Max has taught me how to play cribbage these past few days. Had such a laugh! Well, for starters, he's a cheat and always, well, nearly always wins. Actually, it's a really good game. I shall miss it. Hospital life is... many things: routine for a start, disciplined – lonely, scary, tiring, boring, although I have to say I've barely been bored... barely at all. Well! He's such blooming good company he is. Always pleased to see me – always has some news – always makes me laugh – <u>And</u> he always, well, nearly always is so positive and upbeat and cheerful.

Max Darling, above all, remain "cheerful" – it's your best quality. Besides, there's so many miserable G*ts out there! I'll miss you! Have been so relaxed in myself being here with you – I really have. New heart yes please!!

> *Also, just want to say-*
> *when you're down,*
> *look ahead*
> *when you're blue,*
> *see yellow*
> *when you're sad,*
> *cry*
> *when you're afraid,*
> *look <u>yonder</u>!*

And remember this:- you are strong, very strong (yet we all have moments of weakness) – so, at these times it is when you have to remind yourself of...... The Warrior (Yoga position) –

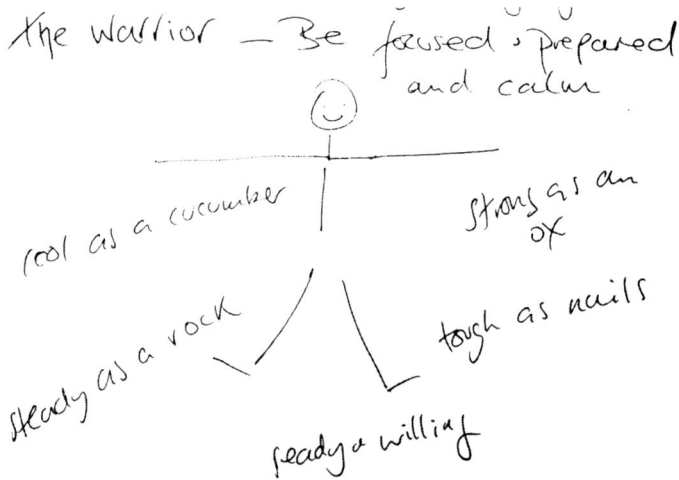

The Warrior — Be focused, prepared
and calm

cool as a cucumber

strong as an ox

steady as a rock

tough as nails

ready & willing

End of Mum's writing

Went to Mum's room for a little snooze after lunch which was really cool – just a change of scenery is enough. Back to my room after that till just before 5 PM, then we went out for a proper walk.

On way out me and Mum bumped into Dr Hasan on the stairs – he is just so committed!! He told us that last night they had an offer on a heart which they thought was going to be good. He said they didn't want to come and bother me until they were more certain, but he said they were excited about it and started to get everything ready (such a nice choice of words – they were excited about it) – they all just so want to see you better here!!

But he said in the end the heart was just not big enough and the donor was H.I.V positive – which apparently is not a deal-breaker when it comes to transplants. So Dr Hasan said he thought it would not be good enough for me.

This may be one of those occasions where the fact that I'm so healthy means that they can be more selective with the hearts – because we've got time to wait for a perfect one. Maybe if I'd have been iller they would have used the heart? Who knows – maybe not?

I have been thinking and talking to Mum about a few things and being here I get the feeling that certainly I, and maybe all of us, do not fully appreciate a few things.

The first is how much risk I am at with my heart. How dangerous it is. The way I understand it is that the right side of my heart barely beats and the left side is inefficient too. That's always been the case but now there are four more real risk factors I think.

One, because my heart just about manages by itself in sinus rhythm, when I have atrial arrhythmias, I go into a greater stage of heart failure. Therefore if my heart gets stuck in a non-dangerous atrial arrhythmia again, like in 2008, I would start to swell and become iller and iller every day with congestive heart failure. And as I arrested on Sotalol I now can no longer be treated by anti-arrhythmic medications easily. So all they could do would be another ablation again, but they said that's very hard.

Second is my ventricle arrhythmia risk – this is why I've got my I.C.D (Internal Cardioverter Defibrillator – an advanced pacemaker) but that's no complete failsafe. My heart could go into a ventricle arrhythmia which would be acutely dangerous – but hopefully my I.C.D would save me because it could happen as quick as my cardiac arrest in September. But they say the I.C.D would only save me when it happens – not stop it happening – so there's a real risk there. That one doesn't bother me too much (touch wood) as I've never had malignant ventricle arrhythmias before, except when on Sotalol and I haven't had one in the year and a half since my arrest, so I think that's not too much of a bad one – but like all rhythm problems it is temporal, so you can be fine for years but that wouldn't diminish the risk.

I think the big dangers of my heart – if I've interpreted the doctors correctly is the small area across my broken prosthetic tricuspid valve. Firstly, blood is flowing very slowly through it as the right side of the heart hardly works and there is probably low pressure around it – this makes the risk of clotting on the valve much, much higher, as the valve is not really moving at all. This I think is the big risk because as soon as you form a blood clot there, well, it's not worth writing about.

The other risk is because the valve is broken and is sort of just flapping about a little half-open, half-closed, it could be that the valve just collapses and then... well again no need to say.

So I think in my general day-to-day life, none of us, least of all me, thinks about all that stuff and therefore, we, by consequence, don't appreciate the actual dangers that are there. And sometimes I think how wonderful it is that we do not appreciate it, because if I did my life would be truly unbearable.

I mean within Newcastle seeing me in June 2009 for a transplant assessment, I am already admitted at The Freeman on the heart transplant list – and they are not doing that without serious just cause.

This leads me onto a few other things that I do not think we fully appreciate; in March 2009 when the Heart Hospital found out my valve was broken and I had my I.C.D implanted the consultant, Shay Cullen, had the frankest talk with me and Pam, explaining the lay of the land.

Mainly, he said that they refer very few of their G.U.C.H (Grown-Ups with Congenital Heart disease) patients for transplantation because of these two main reasons; 1) It is so very hard to get onto the transplant list and; 2) even when on the list is so hard to find a donor and it not be someone sicker who gets it.

Shay said that generally when a heart becomes available, non-congenital heart patients receive it, because of the ease and non-complexity of the operation.

But here in Newcastle these factors didn't matter to them. They put me on the transplant list and then said, in their words, 'that's the least we can do for you. We want to give you the best chance for life...' so they admitted me to the hospital to be monitored and cared for, whilst I waited. Also because the Surgeons are paediatric congenital heart Specialists they have all the experience needed in transplanting the more complicated patients like myself.

So, when I said I've been thinking and talking to Mum about this today – what I mean is, when you take all that in, the risks of my heart and the lengths Newcastle are going to, you do tend to realise how unbelievably lucky I really am.

Day 7 – 06/04/10

Mum left today. Ah bless her, have loved having this time with her. Had a hilarious chat with the cleaner – me, Mum and her – haven't caught her name yet but will – such characters the Geordies – they have a real salt-of-the-earth type quality. Anyway Mum nearly missed her taxi the cleaner was talking so much, but I saw her out and said goodbye outside the Cardiothoracic block.

Then guess what? Guess what I did!!! I played the piano!!! Been thinking for a few days that I should check out the hospital's chapel, because if anywhere there might be a piano it'd be there – I wasn't holding out much hope though. However, as I walked into the chapel there was an upright piano sitting there, with stool, next to the altar.

I walked in and a woman who was part of the chapel staff asked if I was okay and I enquired about the piano. She said of course you can play the piano – please go ahead.

There was only one old lady in there looking at a striped tapestry on the far wall. I started playing and the piano sounded lovely. I played some lovely slow songs – 'I Dreamed a Dream' – Les Miserables and 'All Be Lonely Tonight' and a few others. The old lady came over to me as I started playing 'Bridge over

Troubled Water' and she stood next to me the whole song. When I stopped she said how wonderful it was.

When I first started playing she was studying the embroidered tapestry on the far wall. It was vertical strips of embroidered squares starting in purple from the left and moving through a variety of colours to yellow on the right. It was new and was called the Rainbow. To me it looked an upside-down bar chart whose embroidery in the squares was not delicate or ornate – just the bright colours and simple images like just a circle for the sun and so on.

To me it looked cheap. To me it looked boring – not skilful at all and, I suppose, either a quick patch job for decoration or an arts and crafts project by some school children. It was as unremarkable and as chintzy as you could imagine. But this old lady was studying it for ages whilst I was playing. And when she was talking to me about the chapel she was going on about how beautiful the embroidery really was. She must have been studying it for 10 minutes – it was only small.

I don't really know why I am going on about it so much, but I just think it is so mad when someone finds something genuinely beautiful that I find utterly unremarkable. What is it she is seeing that I can't ? What am I blinded to which she can see there? But the way her face is when she talks about it – she is really impressed. And I think it's just one of those wonderfully simple things of joy. I got a real warm feeling for some reason.

The old lady was really old but still had all her faculties – she was slowly, alone (except for me) in the chapel, admiring it... I don't know, there's just something so right and beautiful in that itself. I don't know if I'm explaining myself properly – I don't think I am. Anyway so good to know I can go and play the piano at any time – am so pleased.

Then Wifey arrived!! Yay. Although when she first walked in we argued – she come into my room from a nightmare train journey and said she was busting for a wee. She went to use my bathroom which is strictly for patients only so I told her to go and use the one outside the ward. She shot me a disgruntled look and stormed off – when she returned her expression had not improved. It's not like the bathroom rules are my rules – I said 'I've got to live here Pam and if they bust you they bust me.' She couldn't seem to understand in her nightmare-journey state, so just glared at me again and sat down in a huff! Nice. We made up a little later though, so no harm done.

Watched the new G.O.S.H fly-on-the-wall series that night. It was all about hearts, Dr Reece (my consultant at G.O.S.H) and surgeon Dr Victor Tsang – my G.U.C.H surgeon at the Heart Hospital – the one who called Dr Hasan to refer me here. Have never seen a program like it. Like it was made for me. Dr Reece looked exactly as I remembered him and still spoke to the child instead of the parent in consultations...... such a wonderful doctor.

I'm not going to write about how the program affected me because I don't want to; save for the fact that it affected me loads. And I suppose made me more scared about my trans-plant. I mean after the surgery I could wake up blind ... or paralysed ... or not at all.

Day 8 – 07/04/10

Woke up in a really down mood. Scared and beaten. I know the programme last night had a lot to do with it, but not sure how much. With feelings you're never sure if the reaction you have is a sole consequence of previous events, or just a single stalk of straw that breaks the camel's back. Either doesn't really matter. I still feel beat.

People say you need to have courage – you need to have resolve, and you need to have fight in you to stay positive – to stay sane – to stay yourself; a happy, outgoing, positive, life-affirming person. You tell yourself this so much, the attributes become easy to portray – even reactionary. They are, quite genuinely, who I am. However, there seems to me a slight grey area which I struggle with.

This positivity, spirit and verve are deep-rooted and feed on the light of hope and faith and happy, positive, jubilant thoughts. However, such roots are scorched by fear. They do not like negativity and despair is like acid, poured, concentrated, over them. Needless to say that it therefore makes for a better psyche, a more peaceful consciousness to do one's best, utmost and endeavour to keep these perils away – like fear, like negativity, like despair. But, and here is the thing, such painful emotions are as important, I think, very, very important to the world – and most of all me. Even though they're so hard to bear.

So, I guess, what I would say, is instead of having the courage and strength to stay positive, have the strength, courage and resolve to be negative – to be scared – to be beat. I guess that's maybe one of the things I've learnt here – but, of course, never one thing too much.

Had nice day with Pam. Taught her Crib which she picked up really, really quickly – although she had no luck at all with the cards and she lost all the time. Went for a walk too after lunch and then had our special prawn pasta in Pam's flat, which was scrummy.

Got back and spoke to a young girl opposite – she is around 25, by herself, having valve replacement surgery tomorrow morning – her first surgery. She is so scared. She is so, so, so, scared. She was in tears as she told me. She has a three-year-old daughter and is petrified of not waking up. I so feel for her – all by herself – in, I reckon, the worst moments of the whole thing (the night before!) She's known since November it needed doing and has been living in fear ever since at receiving any Freeman letter – or private number phone call.

Man, I so think I know what she's going through. I don't really try to comfort her – in such moments comfort is a foreign place – but I do my best anyway. It's like looking in the mirror seeing her fear and hearing her worries. I said to her that the night before is the worst part of all of it – I said tomorrow will be so different. I said after this you'll be free again. But, as I know, such words do not speed up the clock – so nothing has changed.

I had no idea of her circumstances – her dad was in earlier, but now she is alone. And loneliness is not what she needs. I would not be able to do it alone – maybe this is why I feel so much for her – maybe not. I wish her all the best – I must catch her name. All anyone can ever say – be it a Professor of Cardiology or a little child is – 'Good Luck'.

Day 9 – 08/04/10

Talked to the girl opposite last night until about 11 PM – she was okay. Poked my head in her room this morning to wish her the best of luck – apparently she slept a fair bit, only woke at four for a while so that was quite good.

Me and Pam then had my first breakfast trip to the canteen. I had the half Monty – yes please. Pam tells me that Alex has gone through the night again – wonderful – God I miss him. Have been trying my hardest not to think about him – not to look forward to seeing him again, even not to ask about him. I don't really know why – that is why I haven't really written anything about him so far – it is just too hard.

I haven't given myself the pleasure to yearn for him, or picture him, because I don't trust myself to do so. It would just make things so much harder – I mean, well I don't know what I mean. But all I know is the thoughts of Alex tear at me. The thought of him at home and me not being able to see him just defeats me. I miss him so much. But it's not a normal missing, not a normal longing – not like I can describe anyway.

He is my son. He's only seven months old. His tenderness and innocence and purity is amazing – he's like a little bundle of everything that is right in the world, of everything which is good. He is a beacon of joy – he's just so much to me – and I can't see him. And won't be able to for still another week. Another week's torture, unless I try to forget him. It sounds like I'm admitting something bad. I sound heartless saying that I'm trying and do try not to think about him – but if I can't be honest on these pages what's the point in them. I suppose all I can say is that the love I have for Alex is as virginal and pure as he himself – and that this place – this situation – can only pollute that love and for better or worse – whilst I still can – I'll try to keep them apart.

Saw consultant Dr Choudhury, new registrar Mark (his second day) and paediatric nurse Debbie. They talked and joked with me about what I'm reading – about not going for too many fry-ups whilst I'm waiting and about me, supposedly being loaded, because I work in derivatives in the city. Dr Choudhury kept asking what are the best stocks to buy before the election – was quite funny. Didn't have the heart – excuse the pun – to say stocks are equities not derivatives....!

Debbie then said though, after I told her where our house is we are going to rent, that I may be able to go there on a sort of day release and stay there all day – just come back evening, night and morning. Nothing certain yet though, as everything seems to be with hospitals, however would be well, well cool if I can spend the days at our rented house with Alex and Pam and John.

Talking of hospital uncertainties, the young girl's operation was delayed and delayed all through the morning and then cancelled until tomorrow morning. She is in an even more fractious and distressed way now – but she has had her uncle and father with her for most of the day, but it's evening now and she's on her own again. She says if it's cancelled again tomorrow she's going to go home – think that's the fear talking

– at points fear seems to be able to take control of all motor-neural functions!

Her dad couldn't get her TV to work so he came over to enlist my help. When I went in Jessica's room (found out her name) her eyes were red raw and her cheeks rouged with wiping tears. I tried to get her TV to work but I couldn't – think it may be broke. I said to her that nothing is going right for you is it – but it will.

Her dad shook my hand and really thanked me for being there for her last night and apparently making her feel better. Felt really good to be thanked. Can't remember the last time I truly helped a stranger in need – I am wondering if I ever have??? Am sure that whatever help I gave was not some massively altruistic self-sacrifice of mine – just some comforting words of advice from someone who can offer them – however it was probably the most I've ever helped someone I don't know – well knowingly anyway.

Don't know what that says about me or the life I lead. I'm not saying anything is bad or wrong – far from it – it's just when you think about it – or when at least I think about it – truly selfless deeds, helping a common stranger, are hard to come by. The opportunity does just not present itself – either that or in my normal life I do not see such opportunities – the noise of daily living makes people's subtle cries for help unheard – noise which, in the confines of hospital life, doesn't exist.

But whatever I say, I do feel really, really good knowing I've helped – and I really appreciated her dad telling me so. Because her TV didn't work I've leant her my PSP with the first few discs of 24 for her to get into – it's the least I can do. Most of the time my PSP lies unused. Hopefully she'll get done tomorrow morning because she is going through hell inside – although she puts on such a brave face. Bless her.

Watched Liverpool that night against Benfica – Liverpool stormed through to the semi-finals 4-1 however, it's only the UEWAFFA cup, so not really the greatest thing.

That's about it really – turned the TV off and then curled up to go to sleep. Had to have obs done though at about 10:30 – blood pressure was 127/71 temperature 35.8 pulse 55 SATs 100% and respiratory rate 16 – perfect. They would be the readings of an athlete with full health of heart – I still can't believe this all.

Day 10 – 09/04/10

Had just the worst nightmare last night. Was directly about my heart transplant – again I can't remember the details, but was well, well scary. Woke up in a ball of sweat. Surprisingly however, I didn't have much trouble getting back to sleep. So now I'm awake and writing. I wished Jessica good luck again and she gave me back my PSP and I'm just waiting for Pam to … ah that's her calling now – she didn't have a good night – awoke at about 1 AM a little panicky. I told her she should have called me, she dismissed it. She's still in bed and not going to rush. She's going to get up and have breakfast and then come over – where would I be without her?

Will play some Skatt today. You see we have been playing this card game 'Shit-Head'. We learnt it whilst we were travelling and it's a really good game – better if there's a few of you but it's still really good for just two. Anyway we've always said that we've got to come up with another, non-offensive name for it, because if a doctor, or nurse, or indeed anyone casually asks what are you playing, you can't really reply 'Shit-Head' now can you.

So yesterday I said that we should call it Skatt in public – this is because in the book I'm reading – 'All Quiet on the Western Front', the card game the soldiers constantly play is called Skatt. However, Pam is not too keen. She thinks that we should stick to our travelling roots and keep calling it Shit-Head. I don't think she quite realises the difference in social atmospheres between travelling and being at home/hospital.

Travelling no one would bat an eyelid at a game called Shit-Head – I mean most of them know the game anyway, but travelling through hostels and stuff there exists very different social standards and ideals than compared to say in hospital. I mean the sense of hygiene for one are worlds apart – for instance, when travelling it's perfectly acceptable to have a change of smalls once every four days, whilst here it's a maximum of two days!! Or wait, maybe that's just me . . . yeah, I think it probably is.

Anyway where was I? How did I get comparing pant-life-between-washes from travelling to in hospital??? Urmmmm . . . oh yeah . . . Shit-Head – arghh, I mean Skatt – oh sod it, I think you get what I mean; in more common, acquainted and personal company we can carry on calling it Shit-Head – that will keep Pam happy and publicly – or at least to anyone who asks who seems like they'd be offended, or embarrassed by the real name, we'll then call it Skatt. Sorted. Still now comes the problem of identifying if an innocent inquirer about the game falls into the first or second categories. . .

Can you tell I'm bored? I bet you can. Urmm what can I write about to pass a bit of time? Well, writing about what I could do to pass the time actually passed some time itself. And so did that. And that too. . . I feel I'm losing the plot here. . .going around in circles. There must be something constructive I can write about? I know – I can try to make up a hospital joke – like my altered words to the nursery rhyme 'Row row row your boat' – just for the record;

Row, row, row your boat, gently down the Somme,
when you get older, you can tell us, stop singing that stupid song!!

Haha brilliant – now, a hospital joke. Urmmmmmmm. . . what about a 'how many' joke which uses the different classes of nurses as the base stereotype to draw humour – am thinking something like;

How many auxiliary nurses does it take to measure your blood pressure......?

Haven't got a punch-line yet, but was just a for instance ...urmmmm, let me think. What is funny about hospitals? What common ways, which are normal here, would seem funny and strange when singled out from an observation? I've got one, but not sure if it's that funny.

With every set of obs they do they ask you if you're in any pain. Now I always say no, however, if you say yes they ask you to grade the pain you're in by marking yourself on the following scale;

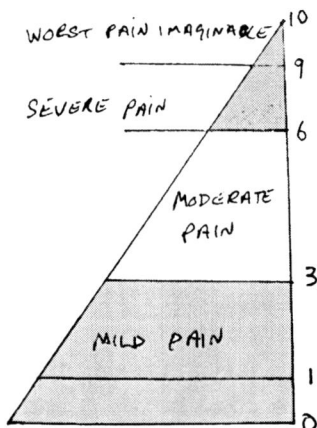

This is the official AVPU pain score that hospitals use and is all quite unremarkable – except for the descriptions of the different pain thresholds – most notably of all 9-10, captioned as 'worst pain imaginable.' It's the 'imaginable' bit that has caught my eye in terms of making a hospital joke – I'm thinking something like this:

Nurse: Are you in much pain sir?
Patient: Argh, ouch, *(pant-pant)* yeah......
Nurse: How much pain would you say you are in on a scale of 1 to 10?

Patient:	*grown, moan, stutter-* ner...ner......nine?
Nurse:	9? So you're in as much pain as someone who has had both of his arms and legs cut off and salt poured on the open wounds – that sounds like the worst pain imaginable...
Patient:	*turns green and shuts up*
Nurse:	So do you want to rethink your score Sir? And please have more respect for the AVPU scale – you've only got a migraine
Patient:	*dumbfounded and confused* – Can I just have some Paracetamols please?

Okay, this is not that funny at all, but it's only a first attempt – I'll keep thinking – have got plenty of time.

Jessica, opposite, was taken down to theatre in the morning – I had my door shut but was so distressing. She had her dad with her, but as soon as the Porters came up to her room she burst out crying. Kept saying she couldn't do it and that she wanted to go home – kept saying 'nore' ('no' in the Geordie accent).

Her dad was softly reassuring her saying it'll be all right, but must have been so upsetting for him – seeing his daughter so, so distressed, as well as the pain of knowing what physically is about to happen as well.

She just sobbed and sobbed all the way down the corridor. They should have given her a stronger pre-med – but what do I know? I think, although not completely sure, she said 'I don't want to die.'

We're all scared of not waking up after surgery. But, sometimes, when I'm alone, and even alone from my conscience, I permit myself to remember something I can barely explain, but something that, nonetheless, on a completely, utterly selfish level, really appeases that fear of not waking up – it's knowing, in a weird sense, what not waking up is really like...

*   *   *

I was playing Scrabble. I was feeling so much better and a three-week illness of suffering from congested heart failure had come to an end. I was on my bed, in The Heart Hospital's ACW Ward, all washed and showered, clean, unswollen – I had my ankles back and my heart rate was finally nice and slow … then … I stirred … a few abstract memories – of an awareness of thought, but not body … a few 'made up images' – for I see them from across the room … the letter 'H' sign languaged … a vague wondering somewhere distant of … What?? What's happened? Again more abstraction … more distance … more disorder of surreal vagueness.

Then, Pam's voice … stronger … a choke of something moving in my throat – unpleasant – but still indifferent. Then, like jumping into iced-water, I was fully awake; aware; lucid – just like that.

Within moments I knew what had happened; 'You had a cardiac arrest Max, yesterday and was resuscitated and brought down here to intensive care … you were playing Scrabble'… Scrabble… SCRABBLE… my mind latches onto the crystal clear memory of that game … sitting on the hospital bed … John in the chair next to me … Pam opposite … just argued about the banking crisis … hair still wet from the shower … my cardiac monitor alarming with 'artifacts'. All instantly so clear, so exact – like the sharp cut of a knife through soft melon flesh – so precise. And in that instant recollection all so … so … so … so … distant.

No-one understands our perception of time and how we feel how close or distant certain events seem to us – so the facts are meaningless: I was unconscious for just over 24 hours.

But SCRABBLE … that Scrabble game … my wet hair and banking crisis discussion – was years ago wasn't it? Months and months ago? Absolutely ages ago? I've been asleep for ages – for a massive amount of time – forever? But now I'm awake. I'm back –

I'm here. That's good isn't it? That's handy. It's nice to be here.

But – and this is the most awful – well perhaps not awful – but most certainly damning thing to life I can admit to – is that, that time – that unquantifiable amount of time between Scrabble and reawaking – well – that was fine. Am pleased to be back here with everyone, but that gap in-between – which for all I knew and felt could have been forever, was okay too. Not bad. Not painful. Nothing much at all. And this is what I'm so ashamed of.

In my dark moments, when I am just so scared of dying, or not waking up after surgery, I placate myself by the feeling I had when I first awoke after my cardiac arrest – that dying – for me – really wouldn't be that bad at all. So, as far as I totally and selfishly am concerned, it doesn't really matter if I die. It's the only way I can quiet my mind. But it's a terrible – shameful – awful thing to admit.

If I don't make it and Alex reads this I would be so sorry for admitting this – so, so, sorry – but I've done it now. My secret is now set in ink – preserved for as long as there is light left in this world to read it. I am truly sorry everyone – Pam and Alex especially – I truly am. I feel like I'm confessing perhaps my deepest crime. But you can be the judge of that.

*   *   *

Didn't see hide nor hair of a doctor or transplant coordinator today – there is nothing they need to come and see me for, however, it is rubbish hanging around your room until mid-day just in case they do come to see you. And it would be nice if one of the transplant team poked their heads in to see how I was doing, I mean it has been a whole week since I've seen any of them. However they may have popped around when I haven't been here so can't judge them too harshly. And I did say I'd shout if I need anything and other than that they needn't worry coming to see me so it's my own fault really. Not that I'm that bothered.

Walked over Paddy Freeman's Park and sat by the lake for quite a bit. The weather was really nice – sunshine with just a little cloud, but no wind. Still needed a light jacket or jumper, but was pleasant to sit outside. We also bought these ginormous cakes from the Italian deli and sat and ate them outside; Mnnnnnnn, they were well nice.

Then me and Pam in the evening snuggled on my bed and watched Great British Menus and some of Harry Potter and the Goblet of Fire – which I think should have been called Harry Potter and the Tri-Wizard Cup. Watched a bit of the U.S Masters then had a good night's sleep.

Day 11 – 10/04/10

It's getting beyond a joke now how much I'm missing Alex. It's really starting to upset me. I had tears in my eyes yesterday when I pictured myself cuddling him again. Was on the phone to Jen and she put the handset next to Alex so I could hear the raspberries he was continuously blowing – sounded like an adult blowing them they were so loud. Could have just cried my eyes out at that too.

Oh man it's just so hard being away from him for all this time. It's been so long since I've scrunched him – so long since I've held him up and played tick-tock with him. So long since I've dressed him, or changed his bum, or fed him, or cared for him. Thursday I get to see him again but today is only Saturday. What utter rubbish! I ache for him. Feel my chest crawl with desire to scrunch him. Get a tingling all over when I think about his adorable face with his gaping smile – it will light up this hospital room more than any eastern facing window on a clear morning.

I can't wait for that feeling of perfection to sweep over me again – into my eyes and ears and finger tips, when I hold him again. I just can't wait to be cured by him soon – not too long now. I. Want. My. Alex. That is what, now, my heart desires the most.

Still mustn't stew too much. Tom is coming to see me today
– yeah!!!!!!!!!!!!!! It's coming up to 8:30 AM so I think he should
be landing in Newcastle around about now if everything is
going to plan, so that is way cool – am looking forward to that.
Oh and the nurse I really get on with well is on today which is
really good because Tom will be able to stay all day without
getting ruled-booked on visiting times.

Was really good timing because Dr Hasan came round at
about 10-ish with another older consultant who I haven't met
before and can't even remember his name – however, he's
come up from working at G.O.S.H for a while.

As always there was nothing medical to discuss so we talked
briefly about Dr Reece, who they both know really well. The older
consultant asked if he'd changed much from the programme – I
said he is just as I remembered him 10 years ago. I said he was like
'Doc' out of 'Back to the Future' where he looks the same in every
decade! They both quite laughed actually.

Anyway Dr Hasan said enjoy the nice weather, so when Tom
turned up 15-20 minutes later I thought I may as well leave my
hospital room for a long stint – I mean it's the weekend and I
just saw the doctors and there's hardly any patients and
therefore nurses, on the ward, so I thought 'sod it'.

Me and Tom left at 10:30 AM and didn't come back to the room
until 3 PM! We watched a football game over the park, I showed
him the chapel and the piano, we went and knocked for Pam at
Beechwood, but she was in the bath. Then for lunch we drove to
Sainsbury's and bought a French stick and lunch stuff, came back
to the hospital and laid out on the grass for a picnic.

Weather was so nice I was even down to my shorts and T-shirt
laying there. Then at 3 PM we went back to the room so they
knew I was still alive and had not done a runner.

We then played some Crib – Tom brought his Crib board
which is really cool and I set the place alight with a 15 point
check out!!!. Pegged 3 points and had a dozen in my hand –
rock on. Tom was stunned, but of course, why wouldn't he be

– it's not often that you see someone finish in the hole from 15 points out – a game to remember that was.

Then a little after 5 PM we drove out and found Tom some digs down Osborne Road and also found a well, well nice Chinese there too, which was well expensive, but well worth it – we had loads and wolfed it down.

On way back to my room after we had all separated – Tom to his hotel and Pam to Beechwood – I saw Jessica's father. He said her operation went really well and she is out of intensive care and on Ward 25 – and that tomorrow she should be up and walking. He said for me to go and see her, which I will definitely do – nothing like seeing a healthy-looking girl go for open heart surgery, coming through, out of ITU and back to health again – to settle my pre-operative nerves.

Will probably go down tomorrow or the day after because it's a very personal thing seeing someone in a hospital bed with wires and hospital gowns on and stuff and I don't want to invade her privacy yet – it is a whole lot easier and subtler when you're more up and about and better.

Watched some more golf and had real trouble getting to sleep. Night times are definitely the worst. I find myself wanting them to come and tell me they have a heart for transplant primarily to relieve the monotony and loneliness of laying awake in a hospital bed, trying to drift off, all alone with only the beeps and alarms of other patients' cardiac monitors for company. Still, after a short while it was morning – announced by my morning obs needing to be done.

Day 12 – 11/04/10

Tom walked over early and got here at about 9-ish. Pam arrived soon after whilst me and Tom were playing crib. Was pleased that Tom got to meet Dr Hasan who came round just before 10, although Tom probably wasn't too bothered to meet him. We talked for a few minutes – Dr Hasan said it was only a social call and then they left. I really think a lot of him coming to see me on a Sunday morning again just to see how I'm getting on – he really must work 6/7 days a week, I'm sure of it.

We walked again and watched some more footy over the field and had a brew by the lake. Played Nominations as you can see opposite [*original journal contained card game scores*] and Pam won. I was docked 10 points for 'accidentally' laying a trump when I had a heart which was the lead suit. I mean a simple honest mistake like that is harsh to be punished so – however it didn't matter in the end – Pam won by quite a bit. She was quite lucky – she'll get me for saying that – to be honest she did play really well to win.

Then we both listened to Tom playing the piano in the chapel. He really is so good. He played and sang his song 'I'm Wondering Why?' I tell you that song holds a beauty and depth which is so very strong. It is so moving. It's like the music is a language that speaks to that deep place inside you which normal sound cannot penetrate. It flows in and down deeper than any swallow and makes a little nest right inside your very core which is as warm as a gently crackling log fire in a wooded wilderness, and as comforting as soft plump cushions, plenti-fully arranged around the glowing embers of that very fire.

That song just does so much to me. And this is the wonder of music I suppose. I've gone on about 'I'm Wondering Why?' But so many songs can get you there – so many songs and scores can sweep over you, prick your neck hairs up and dive down to swish around your soul.

I think music is one of the most wonderful and profoundest of things. I reckon it is summed up best by Albus Dumbledore – the Headmaster of the world famous Hogwarts School of Witchcraft and Wizardry – when he said 'nothing we do here is as magical as music'. How can you say anything more than that?

Then Tom had to leave. Was surprised how sad I was when he

went. Had to hold back tears as I walked back to Pam's digs. Spending time with Tom is like nothing else of compare... I'll leave it at that. Some things words cannot touch.

*   *   *

Am becoming slightly unnerved. Have spent loads of hours away from my room without anyone saying anything, so I know I can spend long periods of time away, out and about. And even when I'm here it doesn't much feel like a hospital – I can have visitors whenever I like and I still do my own meds and I.N.R testing. So it's really, really good and also Pam moves into the house Wednesday (three days time) and Alex (my gorgeous baby Alex) will be moving up and soon I should have my work computer also.

So, I could be able to be away from my hospital room for ages – even though when I'm here it's not really hospital – be at home with Pam and Alex all day, still work and interact with colleagues and go for wonderful walks and meals seeing as The Freeman is in such a lovely spot.

Can you see why I'm becoming slightly unnerved and nervous? Can you see why I am worrying about the oncoming 'good' things?' Because of my opening entry in this journal. I'm scared of changing back worlds and having to go through that chest-scything pain of falling back down into this one again. I'm scared of starting to love this life up here – because if I do that, when the call comes, I'll have to change worlds yet again. And I'm not sure how many more times I can do that – I am really not.

Spoke to Mum before I went to sleep and she says I'll never not be able to change worlds without being able to cope with it. Arh, that gives me some confidence. I suppose that means the answer to how many more times can I cope with it would be 'just once more, as always...'

WEEK **3**

Day 13 – 12/04/10

I awoke to the clearest, bluest morning so far. The sun burning brightly through my window, bringing with it the wonderful morning light, framed in the most perfectly clear blue sky.

When I drew back my blinds the rays of light seemed to flood into my brain, find my thoughts, and make them say – 'it will be okay Max.' I charge anyone to be able to look out of this window, at this morning and not feel hope – not feel content – not feel peace. For such clear light and deep blue can only inspire and comfort. And it has comforted me this morning.

The sky is so clear your thoughts can reach all the way to heaven it seems. At least it feels like that when my face dances in the rays coming down from above – through the glass and into my eyes. On a morning as clear and bright as this, maybe even dad can see me looking out? I asked Mum what dad would have made of all of this if he was still here. We both had trouble answering. We agreed however that dad would have sorted out lots of practical things with much less fuss – getting to and from Newcastle, finding a house to rent, buying certain hospital time-killing gadgets and books – he would have just bought lots of them for me.

But, I suppose, a big thing he would have been able to do is support Mum. Me as well obviously, but I have Pam – Mum doesn't. Still that's just the first few things that came to our minds. On a morning as clear as this perhaps I can ask? But maybe I already know what he will say anyway – it's just that they appear to me as my own thoughts......

Well whatever, the morning is still gorgeous. And I feel not too bad. I keep having this giddy horrible thought though that this could all just go so wrong. But with a morning like this I haven't thought of that since I just wrote it and it's 9:45 AM, so that's good going, I suppose.

Pam has also just arrived bless her. She awoke for hours in the night again. Will be so much easier for her when her dad and Alex are here – feel a little guilty sometimes that I've split them up because I couldn't stay here by myself. But that feeling is fleeting. Hopefully the doctors will come round early so me and Pam can enjoy the sun – we'll see.

Just whilst we are waiting for the doctors to come round I've got to write down the only bug-bear I have with this place with regard to the food … BREAKFAST. My most uninteresting and almost chore-like meal of the day, is made worse by one startling fact; if you tick Weetabix for your cereal you get a packet – which by the way you can never open – of one Weetabix!! One! Can you believe that! Thought breakfast was meant to be one of the really important meals of the day, so can't believe it.

So I started ticking the Weetabix option and then writing next to it 'X2 please'. That worked for a few days and I got two packets, but now even with my extra writing I'm back to just one Weetabix. Ridiculous!

I said to Pam this morning that when they bring my menus round again today, I'm going to write next to the Weetabix option, 'X2 please – my seven month old son has one whole Weetabix and he's only one eighth my size – think a grown adult should qualify for X2'. Well I might write that – if there is enough room on the menu!

And don't even get me started on the little plastic pots of Robinson's jam. How the hell are you meant to open them??? I wish someone could tell me. There's this little pathetic perforated corner which is meant to be able to crack away from the main plastic pot, so then you can peel away the film over the jam. Well... what do you think... you've guessed it – the tiny corner peel back thingy is horse shit – it just doesn't work at all. Every morning I fumble around its stupid perforated edge and do you think that damned thing ever breaks clean and peels back? No. Never. I think I've had one that has worked in two weeks. It's just infuriating. I mean can it really be that hard? Would love to go up to the head of products and packaging at Robinson's, go right up to him, look him in the eye and just shake my head and then walk off. I mean in this day and age.

It reminds me of the time I wanted to write to McVitties to suggest they change their 'tear here' label to 'tear *nowhere near* here'. Oh the stupid little things that annoy you – but they are infuriating!!!

When Amanda and another older consultant came round they pretty much confirmed that I could, in the daytime, if there was nothing planned for me for that day, go to our rented home, just around the corner – how cool is that.

Me and Pam then laid outside pretty much all day. At one point we were by the Lake, drenched in noon-day sun, shorts and T-shirt and ice cream, laying there, listening to the children's hum of activity from the park and wind chimes in the chiming tree and in that moment, we could have been on holiday. The walls and worries of our current situation seemed to have briefly melted away and we both enjoyed empty idle hours together.

Went to see Jessica on Ward 25 – she looked really, really well, although she said she felt terrible. She didn't have any tubes or wires in and looked bright and healthy. She said however that she was in loads of pain with her chest and her back – that she's had hardly any sleep and that she's been sick lots and not been able to eat hardly any food. All that being the case though, Dr Hasan said she may be able to go home tomorrow or the day after – she's just got to be able to blow into this box thing with enough force to make the three balls inside (in inner tubes) go to the top. She could only lift the first one when she tried it, so she needs to heal more to expand her puff.

Still, it's mad how well she looks – just the physical healing of the bone, which is a pain, but nothing more and it's all over for her. I said she's done really well, although she said about shouting out as the porters come, about wanting to go home. She just said it was the worst and hardest moment of her whole life.

She said she would try to pop up and see me before she gets discharged and really thanked me for going to see her. Just another valve replacement patient – admitted, operated, recovered out of I.T.U and now close to going home. As simple as that!

That night when I went to fill up my water I saw Kirsty (transplant coordinator) by the nurses station in full operating scrubs – my heart well skipped a beat, as thought she might be coming to me. I have to admit that in that split second when I saw her look up at me and walk over, my mind said 'no' to itself. I couldn't stop it. It was purely reactionary. What do you think that means?

Perhaps it is a normal instant reaction – like a basic instinct of trying to protect yourself from the danger of surgery. I don't think I should read too much into it – I can only imagine my instant reaction being one of joy if I was really unwell – so I suppose the 'no' means I'm doing well… anyway Kirsty was there because they just flew up a youngish girl for a lung transplant. Again all you can say is 'good luck'. Think the operation went ahead.

Day 14 – 13/04/10

Guess what? Breakfast – I not only got two Weetabix but the jam opened correctly without a hitch as well. Hopefully my transplant will be today because things are already going my way and with two Weetabix and an opening jam pot there's nothing that can stop me now......

Well I've got to try to keep myself sane with little jokes and anecdotes like that, or I don't know what mental state I'll be in. I know I'm losing my heart, so I'll be damned if I'm going to lose my mind also. No way – I refuse to be discouraged, I refuse to be discouraged.

Weather is absolutely rubbish today – could not be in more contrast from yesterday – the grey soup is back. Land and grey – that's all there is out of the window.

Am waiting for Pam and am a little bored. Pam's got my book Icarus in her bag so can't read and TV is rubbish. Too early to go and play the piano and don't want to play my PSP. Shall I write a poem? Yeah – I haven't done that yet have I. Okay here goes;

Mental Malaise
(poem title decided 25/04/10)

I don't know what to write,
I have no use for this pen or this page,
This ink is a waste as to the space it takes up,
For I really do not know what to say.

Everyone asks, bless them, they all want to know,
But they can't, I don't think, they simply can't know,
So why bother trying to explain, why bother at all?
Oh what am I saying – I just don't know.

Well I've read better poems, that's for damn sure,
Perhaps I'll add to this one no more,
Oh I have to say something don't I, at least one thing, surely I can?
Oh what's the use? What's the point? I'm putting down this pen.

Yep, another world beater!! Haha. Actually it's not too bad for a
first attempt – I think I'll call it... I'm not sure... indifference?
No. Abstraction? Possibly. Malaise? Will have to check that word
in the dictionary. I'll come back to it – when decided I'll write
the poem name in black ink.

Docs came round then me and Pam had a real chilled out day –
we were both really knackered and just really chilled out.
Found the Asda and bought some snackage. Then I went to
play the piano for a little, whilst Pam went to my room to watch
another waft cookery show – the TV is littered with them.

As I sat down to play, a man walked in and sat down quietly
by himself, right at the back of the chapel. I gingerly asked if
he would mind me playing and he said in quite a posh accent
"of course not – please go ahead." So I started playing and
after five minutes or so, when I was playing 'Wonderful
Tonight', I heard him just burst into tears and really sob. I
didn't look up. I didn't look over to him. I certainly didn't
stop and ask him if he was alright – I mean of course he
wasn't okay – he was sobbing in a chapel, in a hospital. I knew
I had to keep playing. In a way I felt like that was helping
more than anything I could say or offer.

After a while the crying stopped. He just remained there at
the back – silent – listening – I never once looked up. I didn't
want to intrude. He didn't need my stare, or my concern – I
think he just liked listening.

After about 20 minutes I stopped playing and rose to leave.
He got up also and went out with me. He thanked me for
playing. Said that 'Wonderful Tonight' was the best – that's
when he cried. He must have been mid-40s, well-dressed and

softly spoken. I told him I was an inpatient and came to play the piano whenever I could. He shook my hand and said 'I'm Paul.' I immediately replied 'Max'. He then softly said 'good luck' and really looked into my eyes.

It was like there was so much meaning between us. Like there was a sea of pain and struggle that we could both see each other in, but neither of us needed to say anything. It was that strange sense of oneness – or camaraderie that you can feel in a stranger, instantly, within certain situations. Who knows his battle – who knows anything of his life, or he mine – but in that brief moment, it felt like there was a great spirit between us – a great understanding, although neither of us knew anything of one another.

It's one of those rare moments, I feel, when you really see and touch the human spirit – in all its hope and sadness. We were two strangers before and after – but I felt like we shared a moment which is unique and very special. A moment when you realise the communality between us all – a moment when I realise one of the finest and most beautiful parts of the human condition – kinship. The very heart, perhaps, of the human spirit.

Then he walked off and didn't look back. I'll probably never see or know anymore of him, but that brief moment was – I'm not sure if I'm saying it right – a treasure.

When I got back to the room the nurse knocked on the door and said don't go anywhere because Lynne (transplant coordinator) wants to see you. Pam instantly asked if I was all right because she thought 'this might be it!' But I wasn't too scared because if it was 'it' she would just come straight up and if we weren't there she would call us straight away – so thought that she probably just wanted to see us.

I was right – did you really need to ask? She came up and chatted to us, but primarily she wanted to see if I could go and talk to a family downstairs who have just come up for their transplant assessment. They are looking to follow the same path as me, Lynne said – transplant review with no decision, but a probable active listing next time they come up (between 2-4 weeks), then possible admission.

So it looks very similar and they seemed to be as shocked at the whole thing as we were – the 24-year-old boy Bobby, looks okay, slightly symptomatic though with shortness of breath and apparently he has bad days when he can't do anything hardly, so don't think he has a good quality of life. Certainly not one which he was used to a year or so ago.

He only has one beating chamber and poor tricuspid valve function, so they are weighing up further valve surgery or transplantation – very similar to me.

Bob was there with his girlfriend and Mum and Dad and they all seemed so lovely. I talked to them for about an hour and three quarters – Bob asked lots of questions like, 'do you feel guilty about waiting/hoping for someone to die? Do I ever feel selfish for taking all the attention and making the lives of my loved ones around me harder/less enjoyable? And do you wonder what it would be like to have someone else's heart?' Questions that could only have come from him. And was really pleased he felt comfortable enough to ask them – I know I probably wouldn't have.

I did my best to answer and tell them what it's like for me without censor. About the heart being someone else's I said that things tend to become yours after a while of being inside your own skin. I explained that when I first awoke with my metal tricuspid valve it was really strange; knowing I had a metal object in my heart which ticked as loud as an annoying wrist watch. When going to sleep, when underwater, when all went quiet, I could hear the ticking resonating through the air and also up through my body. It was foreign and strange. Off putting and invading. It was like something alien was inside me which I couldn't get away from.

However, time is the King of healers. And after time I started to get used to it. I started to befriend it. I started to accept it. And after a while I stopped realising I had it. Then, 13 years later when it broke, my heart no longer 'ticked'. And it actually felt like I had lost something – like something of mine had been taken away. And that's what I hope it will be like with a donor heart. At first it will be strange and foreign and someone else's, but hopefully, like my St-Jude prosthetic tricuspid valve and Metronic I.C.D (pacemaker), it will become me – a make up of my identity – a part of who "I" am. That's what I'm hoping.

Anyway they really thanked me for talking to them and I left them my name and mobile number if Bob wanted to call or text. They said they'll see me when they come up again in about a month's time. They wished me all the best of luck, bless them.

Then watched G.O.S.H series and went to bed. Took me ages to get to sleep but wasn't tossing and turning. I was comfortable and did eventually drift off, '...To sleep... perchance to dream ...'

Day 15 – 14/04/2010

Yay, Pam moves in today!! Woohoo. She's just gone to pick up the keys. I'm going to give the doctors until about 11 to come round and then go over to the house to knock for Pam – haha, how cool does that sound!

*   *   *

It's 9:40 PM and am a bit tired so will be clinical and austere in my diary for today's events. Went to the actual transplant office and saw Lynne – she'd been up all night from when we saw her yesterday afternoon – she'd been setting up a heart transplant for a seven month old on the urgent heart transplant list. She thanked me for seeing Bobby yesterday and gave me a laptop with a heart transplant presentation on it. The transplant office was a hive of activity with files, papers, maps, and phones everywhere.

Then went to the house – met Pam and the inventory clerk there. The house is perfect. Extremely clean, loads of space, nice furniture and a real good feel to it. Kev and John arrived and we unloaded all our stuff and the place already looks like home. Kev then got straight back in the van to drive back home – he's done so much – gone to such effort for us. I am so grateful. And John – well, I can't begin to explain all he has done and will do for us.

Got two really nice messages today. One text from Bobby's Mum and a note from Jessica;

Bobby's Mum's Text

'Hi. Hope you are ok. Just wanted to say thank you for taking the time to talk to us yesterday it meant so much. We hope you get a heart real soon and wish you happiness for u and your family's future. Thanx again. Sheree – Bobby's Mum x'

What a wonderful text. I'm telling you there are few feelings like it when you learn that you have truly and genuinely helped someone. It almost feels like a great privilege – almost like you're the one receiving the gift. And then when I got back from the house after we had dinner there, at about 8-ish, there was a note in my room to me from Jessica;

Note from Jessica

Just want to say good luck and thank you for your support, please keep in touch, thank you, Jessica.

I feel so proud of these two things – I really do. It's just such an excellent feeling when you've helped, you've contributed, you've given. . . it really is something. Well think it's time for an episode of 24 and bed... Alex tomorrow! I get to be with my son again – again, if it were I could fly.

Day 16 – 15/04/2010

Last night I read through the laptop program Lynne gave me about heart transplants. It was a very sobering read. You realise that a heart transplant is really an ongoing, constantly monitored treatment – not a cure. There's so much stuff that can/might happen.

Have to take loads of tablets which have side-effects and then you need to take tablets to counter those side-effects. Rejection is always a threat. Grade 1, 2 or 3 (severe) – most of the time meds need changing, but it will be trips to Newcastle to do so. Immunity is lowered so you can catch things easier, be re-infected by viruses already living in you – like chickenpox, Mumps, polio and others. Also increases risk of cancer – especially skin cancer. You're not really advised to go in the sun, and if you do, you should wear a factor 30 or above. You'll have to monitor your weight, temperature and blood pressure daily as these are early warning signs of rejection – you should keep a chart on all three. I may be readmitted to hospital to deal with rejection at any time no matter how many years after transplant.

Chronic rejection is a very slow rejection over time and is little understood. The only fix is re-transplantation whose results are not great. The medicine can make you forgetful, contract things like cataracts and glaucoma, lead to osteoporosis or problems with bone strength – can give you digestive problems and stomach ulcers and stuff. Long-term medicine side-effects can damage your kidneys so badly that some people even need kidney transplants as well.

If you get ill, feel fever, vomit, have any strange symptoms you have to phone the transplant team. Before taking any other medication, even over-the-counter stuff you have to phone the transplant team. You will have quarterly blood tests and then semi-annual biopsies. You're meant to keep a high-level of hygiene and wash hands all the time and keep kitchen and stuff clean. And that's hardly the half of it! Still there are benefits too... but it's such a big thing. One of the people, however, featured in the presentation still plays rugby after transplant – how mad is that.

Well just woke up and have text from Louise saying flight has been cancelled. All flights to Newcastle and any further north are cancelled because of an ash cloud from an Icelandic volcanic eruption. Mum was really upset and crying, however they soon grouped together and came up with a new plan – they are driving up. Mum, Alex and Lou are en route now and are expected here between 10.30-11 AM, as they have to stop a little bit more for Alex apparently, so hopefully it will not have mattered too much, but must have been stressful for them in the early hours of this morning.

An older lady opposite has just been taken down to theatre for valve replacement surgery. The porters came for her and she got on the trolley chatting away about nothing at all important. Saying thank you to the nurse and saying goodbye to what looked like her older son. You would have thought she was being taken for a haircut, or a short scenic drive, by her manner and the way she was acting. Who knows though, perhaps she is 10 times more scared than Jessica – it's just that she's not showing it. Perhaps not – but you just can't know. The way you act on the outside can bear no resemblance to what you're feeling inside – who knows how scared she is? Even though she didn't seem it.

*　　*　　*

Mum, Lou and Alex pulled up outside the house at about 11:30 AM. I just raced out the door – shoes, who gives a damn about shoes – and there was Alex, in the back, in the car seat, just there, my son, sitting right before me. He. Is. Here. The wait is over.

I gathered him up, Pam next to me and gave him a hug. He smiled – his gaping wide jaw smile – like a melon with a large slice removed. God that cuddle was lovely. I took him inside and me and Pam sat with him – of course Alex couldn't stop looking and smiling at Pam, but I can excuse that – she's missed him terribly as well. But I just couldn't take my eyes off him. Oh it was like I was meeting him for the first time. Almost like I'd never seen him before, although he surprisingly hasn't changed much.

Man he is wonderful. I realise now how incomplete I was up here – you know Alex is just the most amazing thing. My son. Ooo I just love saying and writing that: My son Alex. He is my son. My child. My baby boy Alex ... 'Where art thou Alex, for nothing can be ill if he be here ...' bless him.

After a few more days of being quenched and rehydrated by Alex, I'll be ready – the surgeon can have me. With Pam and Alex here I am now fully fuelled and satisfied – the anaesthetist can take me down, for I am all set. With my family here and by my side, I can face anything. I didn't realise how much of a team us three are until today – until now – until I started writing these words. Kirsty, Lynne, Dr Hasan – any of them can come and knock on my door right now – for I am whole again.

Oh Alex is just so cute. Oh and guess what, I almost forgot to write about it – I was too busy being sentimental and deep, but guess what – Alex, only today, has started rolling over at will!!! Can you believe it? All the time we've been apart, all the time that has passed since he first rolled over, more accidentally I think, about a month ago and he chooses today to become fully accomplished at rolling back to front – I mean it's just amazing. He did it three or four times in about 20 minutes and John is sure that he hasn't rolled over since he's had him – except once when he wasn't looking. It's almost like he was saving it until I could see him again. Almost like he wanted me to see it first hand. I got tears in my eyes when he kept doing it. The simplest things are just the most wonderful to witness. It's just been such a wonderful day.

*   *   *

It's nearly midnight and I've just turned the light back on. Have been trying to get to sleep for an hour, but have so many things rushing through my mind; Tom's song, 'I'm Wondering Why', his letter, the transplant office, little Alex's brilliant rolling, long-term chronic rejection, neurology units with donor liaisons buzzing around them, the fancy for a hot cooked breakfast tomorrow, the nurses and doctors meeting and loving Alex, running around the lake without the immediate onset of leaden limbs, being wheeled to anaesthetist's room, chest drains and gastric tubes, a lovely new house, Tom's song again, Dr Hasan, Alex, Pam, the lovely Chinese, the thought of a knock on the door now, the damn light from the corridor, another alarm in the hallway, footsteps, Louise and Mum meeting the doctors, Alex again, his two bottom front teeth, I'm Wondering Why, Pam.........

A cacophony of white noise. A cascade of thought. A mumble-jumble of grey matter. A man, lying in a hospital bed, awaiting a heart transplant, but before that, awaiting the onset of sleep. But it hasn't taken me yet. I'm going to put my pen down, light off and give it another go. My eyes are tired, but my brain is just not submitting...but I'll keep trying – I refuse to be discouraged.

Day 17 – 16/04/2010

I surprisingly got to sleep quite quickly after turning the lights off again which was good and also didn't have any nightmares either, so another bonus. Must fill you in on a few more things yesterday however.

In the morning Asif (Dr Hasan) and Debbie came around on their morning rounds and apparently they (Newcastle) have done four heart transplants in the last four days – they've transplanted one every day. That amount is unprecedented as they usually transplant around one a week, so four in the previous four days is really a lot. I asked Dr Hasan how they all went and he just said 'fine – no problems'. Then he said that they haven't lost anyone in transplant for ages – he leaned over and touched my wooden door though, so as not to tempt fate, which was nice. He said the Freeman has the best heart transplant record in the whole world – that's why it's the world's leading centre. So that is really reassuring, although again in those last moments in the anaesthetist's room, before I go under, I'm sure that won't count for anything with regards to my fear – but I don't know, maybe it will.

Anyhow showed Louise my hospital room – she has no sense of protocol at all! She has a bad back, so when we bowled into my room she laid down on my bed – which is not really allowed – but then she surpassed that by putting her feet and her shoes up on the bed also – which wouldn't even be allowed at home, let alone in hospital!

I said 'get your feet down Louise', no respect these days! I also showed her the chapel and the flats where Pam had been staying. We were walking along the corridor and she got out her bloody camera and kept trying to take photos of me – is she for real?? Typical Louise – goodness knows what everyone else was thinking seeing us walking along, amid a torrent of paparazzi-styled flash photography, past the Medical Physics department and Musculo-skeletal unit!!

That night me, Mum and Lou went to the Chinese again which me, Tom and Pam went to. Man is it nice or what? We ordered pretty much the same things from when I was there last and it was just as nice. Mmmmnnnn just so nice!

Then, at about 8-ish, when I was walking back to my ward I saw Dr Hasan, slowly strolling the other way in normal clothes – going home no doubt, probably an early night for him – although the nurses do say that he sleeps at the hospital quite a bit – he's just so committed. Very briefly spoke to him – he's a really nice, friendly man.

So that's the few things I needed to fill you in on from yesterday. Today I am awake and just slobbing around. Need to have a shower and do my blood and want to have that done by the time Mum and Lou get here at about 9:30-ish. But it's only 8:15 so still have time to slob and indulge my journal!

The morning is reaching to heaven again – so blue and clear and bright. I put on my i-Pod and leant against the window, looking out, listening to 'Times Like These' by the Foo Fighters. Such a tune. All my hairs down my legs and arms pricked up with goosebumps – '*it's times like these we learn to live again......*' such a wonderful song, such a wonderful morning – I could die right here now and be happy, I honestly could.

Am now showered and have done my blood and am awaiting the imminent arrival of Mum and Lulu. Because of volcanic ash in the upper atmosphere due to the Icelandic volcanic eruption, all UK airspace has been closed by N.A.T.S (National Air Traffic Service) so, I'm not sure, but I reckon transplants will be affected too, due to the flying around of the organs?

* * *

Just back in room now and on my own – Mum and Lou have just left. Had the most wonderful of days. Doctors came round early at about 9.30 – Massimo, the other congenital heart surgeon came round for the first time. Then we left my room, say at about 10, and did not return until 7:30 PM. And no one has batted an eyelid at it!

Me and John sorted out his I.N.R testing with the help of Amanda, the paediatric nurse and then me and Mum and Alex and Lou spent the bulk of the day laying out by the lake, drenched in rich sunshine. Alex was adorable – he loved it sitting outside with a vest wrapped around his head as a makeshift sun hat. He looked like a baby Sikh with a turban on – oh he was so cute. Then Pam and John joined us with a proper sun hat for him.

We stayed outside from about 11 until 3 PM. Then went back to the house and Mum cooked us five a lovely chicken roast dinner. Was really nice – the only small complaint I had was that the Cauliflower Cheese was a bit of a trading standards hazard – I mean that there was just hardly any cheese sauce and that is, unsurprisingly, my most favourite part! It should have just been called Cauliflower, then I wouldn't have expected anything more and would have enjoyed it, without moaning about it here – honestly the dinner was lovely though. But this expectation thing is just so critical I think nowadays.

I mean, so many things we judge, not on the merits of themselves, but what we were actually expecting. I suppose this is all really obvious, so I don't really know why I'm writing about it. But sometimes I think that the reason I'm finding it so okay here, so far, is because I expected far worse.

When they said about living here, they said that I probably wouldn't really be allowed out and that I am not guaranteed my own room and that they weren't even sure about visiting hours on whichever ward I was admitted to. But, compare that to what it's actually been like here and this feels like the 'Life of Riley'. But that's only because I expected far worse. If, from my normal life, this world here now was thrust upon me, then I may be, by now, majorly depressed – what with being away from home, normal routine, friends, family, work and so on. So, so, much of what I feel depends on my expectations of things. Maybe that's why it's so hard to find the true and real meaning, or worth of things, because our judgement is clouded so deeply by all our expectations – by all our history, by all our previous experiences which have passed.

It is so, so, so hard – perhaps even impossible – to see things for what they truly are, because it is so hard to separate ourselves from these constant impinging expectations. I'm not really sure what I'm even getting at here, or why I'm getting at whatever it is – perhaps it's just another time-filling journal indulgence – perhaps not.

For when anyone says something is bad or good they are really saying more about what their expectations are, built from their past, than they are anything else. What I'm trying to get at is that sometimes it's hard knowing that you cannot really know the worth and value of things.

Once I argued with my aunt that she couldn't possibly appreciate being able to see every day and not be blind. But she swore blind – excuse the deliberate pun – that she could. But that's just it. Marilyn expects to be able to see – so she therefore cannot know the true worth of vision. I know I can't possibly appreciate it.

And again, this is another part of it – for our appreciation of things is as dynamic and fleeting as the prevailing winds. All of this is so changeable and corruptible and rendering. Something you barely blink at one day, can move your world like a train the next. And through it all, our expectations and judgements of things constantly morph and merge and multiply. That's why it can be so hard sometimes to draw permanence, or a solid grounding in life.

With the worth of all things and perceptions of them constantly in flux, I can find myself sometimes reaching out – far out – to find something solid and steady to hold onto. And the pillar I find when I stretch out, is the love and bond between me and Pam.

Okay, you know we are deeply in love, are married, have a family – be it only small, just Alex so far – and that we mean the world to each other, but there is something far, far greater going on – I'm sure of it. I know so many people have been and are in love, and some couples' bond is so deep it finds another dimension, under the ones the rest of us see. But even this is not what I mean when I think about mine and Pam's bond. It really is something different altogether. Love, Soulmates, each others *raison d'etre* – all do not explain it. With me and Pam it's… it's… well that's just it – I have not a single clue, not an escaping hope, of how to finish that sentence.

You see life spins and twirls, the furniture constantly gets rearranged, the garden re-landscaped and then you move house altogether and around on the Waltzer you go again. There are certain things that remain constant – very deep things, like your centre, your bonds, your cornerstone I've gone on about before. But this isn't good enough, still, to explain me and Pam.

Well I'm not going to get anywhere here trying to explain what is between me and Pam, so I'll stop right now. But I can tell you that what is between us, is as stark here, as it is at home, on a normal, unremarkable day.

I do just love writing about her though. These white-washed walls and sterilised floors melt away when I do and I feel the cradle of her love hold me in a way that makes me know it will never let me go.

Day 18 – 17/04/2010

Think I got to sleep the quickest I have since I've been here last night. It wasn't instantly – not by a long way – but didn't take hours like usual. And slept really well all the way through 'til morning. Had a nightmare, however, about getting called for transplant and then it getting called off, but I suppose that's a reality – not a nightmare!

I wonder when the time will finally come? I wonder when I will literally be taken down to theatre to bring the curtain up on this highly awaited, greatly anticipated show? I wonder when this time will come to bear? It's so hard not knowing – but would also be so hard knowing, so you're damned if you do and, well, you know the saying.

It just could be any time at all, whatsoever. No matter when, I can be called for the fight of my life – quite literally. A great quote Emma told me years ago rings so true here. I had to call her up for the full quote, because my memory is nowhere near as sharp as hers;

Quote:

> 'we must all be ready, somehow, to toil, to suffer, to die. And yours is not the less noble because no drum beats for you when you go into your daily battlefield – and no crowds shout about your coming when you return from your daily victories or defeats.'

It's the, 'we must all be ready...' that gets me. For any one of us can get called at any time – ok, perhaps not for transplant, but for a battle certainly. For a fight for survival, for life, even for sanity itself.

Sister Louise's writing

> I am about to leave here, leave Maxy. My darling, <u>younger</u> brother – the baby of the family. Could it not, Jesus, have ever been the <u>other</u> way around? I-e. couldn't it have been <u>me</u>, the <u>oldest</u>? (Wisest?! Strongest?! Maturist?!) Why the <u>baby</u>? Why the youngest, smallest, weakest(?!) Innocent-ist?! This has always been the way it is, this has always been the <u>norm</u>. Max, my younger brother, has a heart problem, yes, he was born with it, yes, I know, it's terrible, oh well lately It's enlarged / got worse / valve's stopped / swelled up / got tireder / so weak / what can they do? / Ablation? / Medication / monitoring?

Newcastle? Oh – so you can – oh – ok, what does a transplant entail? 10/15 years? Oh – ok sounds <u>ok</u>, I guess...... all the endless, <u>endless</u> questions, answers, worries, discussions, tears & smiles... all of it, <u>all</u> of this <u>SHIT</u> (sorry Mum S**T), why couldn't it have been me...... :-(

End of Louise's writing

Just been speaking to the really nice nurse – I really should catch her name – she's so nice. Probably a little older than me, but someone who is instantly right on my level. Like when you meet someone and first start speaking to them, you very quickly become incredibly relaxed and at home – almost like old friends. It's very similar to the ACW nurse Emma at the Heart Hospital – some people you just instantly gel with.

Anyway, I was talking to her about waiting and how pleased I am that I'm allowed out on day release and that I was initially surprised, because the doctors said that the other people they have done this for have not really been allowed out of hospital. She said that that is because they have never had anyone in on the heart transplant list that is externally so well.

She said she was talking to the transplant team about me, because she hasn't been on the heart ward for too long and she wanted to know what the situation was – think she's a type of nurse manager, so needs to know about the patients on her ward. Anyway she said the transplant team have never had someone like me before. They said he is extremely ill on the inside – that my heart is extremely poorly and therefore is on the transplant list – however on the outside I am extremely well.

The transplant team said to her that they have never seen anyone so well with such a poorly heart. There you have it. That's how much of an 'anomaly' – the phrase the transplant team specifically used – I am.

I've been told many times that it is amazing how well I am. It seems really to be a miracle that I am sitting here writing at all, let alone sitting here mostly asymptomatic. The professors and consultants at the Heart Hospital and doctors here at the Freeman – the world's leading heart transplant unit, can all, it seems, not understand why I am so well.

Why am I so well? Why is it that my heart is extremely sick and yet my body is not? I don't understand it. It's not just one thing I've sneaked through whilst luckily remaining well, it's a whole host of things... further dilation of the right side of my heart, paroxysmal supra-ventricular tachycardia, V.F cardiac arrest, C.P.R and the biggest change of all, my tricuspid valve broke – the valve doors fixed open, creating a natural passive flow of blood through the right side. Regurgitation – blood that shoots back the wrong way when the right side of the heart beats – changed from slight – which is normal with a mechanical valve, as the blood pushes the valve doors closed, which means that some gets through before it slams shut – it changed from slight, to 30% regurgitation. That means 30% of the blood flow goes back out of the heart the wrong way – back down to the liver, instead of round to the lungs for oxygenating. And yet, from slight regurgitation to severe regurge, I still remain well on the outside – I still remain asymptomatic!

Why? Why is this so? Through all that's changed for the worse, through all that deterioration, I remain well. I remain the same as always – I remain just Max. I can't understand it. None of us can, but sometimes I think there must be a reason to it, there must be a point to it all. Sometimes it seems that just too many things have happened, which my body has still tolerated, for it to just be a random anomaly ... Oh I don't know, it's just that I can't help but think there is some destiny set for me – some purpose, or reason there for me in the future – something I'm meant to be here, or well for?

I don't even believe in divinity, or fate really, but when I hear what the nurses and doctors say, and when you look back at my recent history, you just can't help but feel a very slight murmur of providence purveying my life. And although this is unquestionably a good thing, it makes things so much harder in some ways.

You see there is such a paradox we are all facing. Me, but also Pam and my family. I am the same old Max, with my same good-old quality of life, however, inside I have become critically ill and very, very sick – fatally so. Yet there isn't anything for our five senses to hold onto, other than good-old Max. My illness, my sickness, is, invisible. It's completely undetectable by us – nothing more than a phantom who stalks our nightmares, more than our reality. But reality it is.

I am, at this very moment, extremely unwell. This is the crux of the paradox for us all, for how can you understand or innately believe something like this? This is why it's so much harder. Look back a few pages to all the surgical, short, medium and long-term risks of heart transplantation therapy. They are terrifying. They are awful. But they are judged by us in unrealistic terms. There is a huge disconnect between how well I seem, to how well I am – and it is this disconnect that hinders our judgements of the heart transplant risks and fears. We do not, deep down, think I am that bad, so the rigours and perils of heart transplantation seem so bad, so awful. But they really, really are and unfortunately will remain, misconceived.

The problem is we think we are in a bright, light room, looking into a dark, bleak, basement – when really, we are already in that basement – I just hope that it's not as dark as it seems from the bright room above – at least not after your pupils – your perception – have readjusted to the light. I'm hoping it will be something like, 'you know, it's not as dark as you think down here…' Well that's what I'm hoping anyway, because any time now I've got to leave this room – misconceived or not, for that basement… but maybe it won't be that bad. Hopefully I'll be around, in due course, to tell you… hopefully.

*   *   *

It was sad to see Mum and Lou go in the morning. Mum was quite teary as I really don't think she likes leaving me. She's so proud of me you know. She keeps telling me how astounded she is with my calmness and how okay I am up here. Think she's just so pleased her son is doing ok up here, in hospital, all this way from home. She's so happy that I am doing so well, I get the sense that her tears are partly tears of happiness for her youngest son, as well as tears of loving. She sent me a text saying how confident and strong and at ease I looked up here . . . bless her.

Think also that's why she was so upset leaving – because being here you can't help but be reassured, by me, by the hospital, by its wonderful staff. And leaving, almost makes it harder for her, because she's not physically here. Well that's what I guess, but I could be quite wrong!

After they left me, John, Alex and Pam, all four of us, cruised back to the house and spent the day there. Went to Sainsbury's and back and had a nice bath at the house.

Day 19 – 18/04/2010

Airspace is still closed across the UK, due to the volcanic ash, therefore it's looking quite likely that Dan and Emma will have to drive up tomorrow. Emma said that because she's now getting her head around it, she's not too bothered, but will have to wait and see. Other than that I'm just washed and dressed and waiting to see if anyone comes to see me this morning before I put this hospital to my rudder and head for my new-Newcastle home! Think I'll read my, 'Lord of the Flies' book that Lulu bought me whilst I wait – William Golding yes please. . .!

Went to the house at about 11:30 as no one came around. Then us four walked back to the hospital to get the cards to play Nomi-nations and we saw Dr Hasan – nice that he got to meet Alex. He was in shorts and T-shirt and heading into the staff gym. He told us about how he used to play badminton, but has now got a bad knee! He just seems like an ordinary man, who is a friendly casual acquaintance – not the most experienced and accomplished congenital heart surgeon in the country and probably, hopefully, the man who is going to cut out my heart!

*　*　*

Had nice relaxing day and am now back in room. I cooked my special prawn and leek risotto for dinner and we all wolfed it down. Was really nice. Well looking forward to Dan and Emma coming up tomorrow. They are going to drive up as flights are still cancelled. It's pretty mental really. All distribution – all UK and a lot of western Europe's flights grounded. The world has never seen anything like this before and no one knows how long it's going to go on for.

Don't want to write too much today. I don't feel like sharing anything with you except, with Tom's permission – which I have got – I'll share the letter he wrote to me. People may read this journal and think, amongst certain things, that I am wise and insightful – well, if I am, I am far, far, far surpassed by my older brother – and pleased to be so too, for if I wasn't, I would not have learnt and understood anywhere near as much as I do today, which I have shown through my journal. Tom is, without a doubt, my guide. I guess that's all I really need to say.

Tom's letter

Dear Max   *13/04/10*

My body is buzzing with feeling as I write this. As I crawl from place to place, I find things so overwhelming. I thought you might like the lyrics and music to those two songs, so I have put them with this letter.

Max, you know that I feel you are the only person who believes in me when it comes to writing songs? I wonder if you know what it's like when someone believes in you, like you do in me? It gives me so much strength, and it's great to know that these are great for someone. Yes, I do not think you realise how much it means to me.

I well enjoyed coming up to Newcastle the weekend. So, so special. Times like those always are. To be oneself with someone, to sit and feel like you could sit forever.

In my song, 'I'm Wondering Why', although you must never take the total song too seriously, the second verse is so perfect for me. I feel it really is an insight into myself, condensed into four lines

[2nd Verse – not in original letter: 'No I could read a thousand books and still never be sure/Or I could spend my life in thought like thousands have before/But sitting by this fire I'm aware of something more/It's nothing I can share with you, but something I just can't ignore.']

You know, it's been fascinating doing my counselling course, some of the things I have written through it are amazing. I don't know why I say this, but I guess I want to share what I am with you.

I really wanted to take a picture of you & Pam, when you were walking in front of me, arms around each other. I got an overwhelming sense of beauty, just in that moment.

Anyway, I look forward to seeing you again soon.

All the best
Love
Tom
PS mercy!

End of Tom's letter

WEEK 4

Day 20 – 19/04/2010

Met up with Em and Legsy [Dan's nickname] at 11, at the house. I showed them the hospital and the chapel and so on with my normal guided tour. We then went back to the house and had some lunch and watched Disclosure. Then me, Em, Legsy, Pam and John all played Nominations. Was an excellent game, even though I done terribly. Pam won on the last hand – pipped her dad to the post. Then me, Em and Legsy went to the Chinese again – they probably recognise me in there now! Was well nice.

Have just got back and am back in my room alone again. By the way think Emma was quite drunk in the end, as they left me at the hospital to walk back to the house – she does like her wine! It's so lovely seeing them, because originally I didn't think that they were going to come up until after their wedding, which is soon. It's so lovely that in my first three weeks being here, each one of my three siblings have come to see me separately and spent quality time with me.

Also Jen texts and calls to see how I am, auntie Carol has text me – John Fromant left me a voicemail, I got a couple of 'Thinking of You' cards from auntie Jackie and cousin Gina, lots of my friends have phoned me to check how I'm getting on: Vale, Tom, Eddie, Dan, Tobin and Trianda. Paul and Craig called

me from work to see how I'm doing and of course also to sort
out my damned computer, which the I.T department still
haven't fitted with a dongle! Also Syed, Jena and Katz have all
text me from work to see how I'm doing at different points.

There are just so many people supporting and holding me
– it is the most privileged feeling in the world, to know so
many people, so many non-blood and non-obligated people
care so, so much. It is almost overwhelming – like I cannot
take it all on board, because it is just too much. I don't know
if I'm going to make sense here, but sometimes I find myself
trying to ignore, or deliberately un-appreciate the things
people do for me – like when Linda made me a chocolate
cake, but after realising I liked her cupcakes the most, went
home and baked some there and then – like when Donna and
Jane bought me some clothes to come up here with – like
Kevin driving all our stuff up and going back again and uncle
Dave agreeing to drive Mum up here when it's time for the
operation, no matter if it's day, or night.

It's just so lovely all these things. It's so moving to know how
many people care and how much effort they are prepared to
spend for my glory only. I was going to write here about a deed
one of Pam's family offered in private, which was one of the
nicest things, however, out of respect to them, it is proper to
leave it as private – but, nonetheless, the sentiment remains in
this journal – such a wonderful thing it was.

The thing is though, it is so overwhelming, that it makes me feel
kind of like... guilty. Because I want to say thank you, I want to let
them know how much they are helping and how much it means
to me, but I can't. I can't make them appreciate what it's like to be
held by such caring, constant hands. I can't tell them of the
warmth that bubbles up from inside me when I hear of the
lengths and means people are going to, to help. I can't tell them
the personal hope and feeling that this support gives me. It has
such a vivid and vibrant power that it pains me to know I can't
return the sentiment of how much it all truly means.

The phrase 'thank-you' is almost an insult, it feels like, when I say it, but I know, ultimately, that's all I can do. That is why sometimes I try to ignore it, or try to shut out how much this means to me, because it makes me see the void of gratitude I want to fill in return, but just do not know how to. I guess it's something I will have to learn to live with. Throughout my recent years people have helped and supported me and my family to what feels like the ends of the earth, to the very edge of life. And not only can I never hope to repay them, I can never really hope to show them what they have all done for me – family, friends, work friends old and new, neighbours and friends of the family and too many more to mention.

This Journal's testament, if it has one at all, will be the amount that has been given to me by all that have helped and supported me. It makes you realise how much life is worth and how much it is worth living.

Day 21 – 20/04/2010

Three weeks exactly I've been waking up in this bed – in Cubicle 5, on Ward 30, on level 4 of the Cardiothoracic block, at the Freeman Hospital, in Newcastle upon Tyne. Three weeks and no transplant and no false alarms either. But, honestly, it doesn't seem like three weeks. It feels like far, far less. I mean there has been so much going on, what with organising every-thing, visitors, acclimatising to a new way of life and settling in. Honestly, these three weeks feel like a sort of blur.

However, I get the sense that now things have just settled down and I can start to sink into a simpler, more routined way of life. It looks like my routine is going to be to wait for the doctors to come around in the morning, or if they don't, give them to say 11 AM to do so, then cruise to the house and stay with Pam and John and Alex until 8/8:30 PM and then come back here. The only difference will be when I get my computer back I'll be working from hospital in the morning and from home in the afternoon.

There. Set. All in order and organised and now all ready. That's why these three weeks have been such a blur – they have been constantly in flux and now everything seems calm and collected and docile. You watch Lynne, or Kirsty will come round in the next few sentences now I have tempted fate – and life will be back, again, on the waltzer, with no order or stillness. No matter how well it all goes, that's still a certainty. Still, until then, I will, if I can, enjoy the relative quiet time that has descended over my days here, very recently.

Saw Emma and Legsy briefly for a cup of tea in the canteen in the morning and then walked back to the house and said goodbye to them. Had lovely time with them and they me too I think. Then in the daytime us four drove into Newcastle and had a little wander around, then came back and John made Spag-Bol with garlic toast. Mmmnn, was well, well nice. John is just amazing you know. And I need to tell him how so, so here goes

Letter written to John

John

I need to tell you how grateful I am. I need to tell you how much you have helped and are helping me. Any direct help you give to Pam, or Alex, is, as I'm sure you know, help given to me also. I believe, although you may not, that your blood obligation to Pam, does in no way detract from the value of your help and support. I have heard you say 'anyone would do it for their child', almost as a way of absolving yourself from gratitude, or applaud. Whilst this may be how you see it, I do not. I see a father, grandfather and a father-in-law, almost single-handedly keeping my small family practically afloat – with the wheels still going round.

I witness your acute kindness and love to my son, me and obviously Pam. I learn a lot from you John, and not just of things from the past, that you were around for, but how to be respectful and easy-going – two properties I would do well to learn from you John.

But the help, the support, the refuge you have given and shown me John I am so, so grateful for. And although you may not want my gratitude, I'm going to give it anyways.

John, I'm so pleased you're up here with me. I'm so pleased there is someone, like yourself, who can be there for Pam and Alex whilst I'm confined in here. I'm just so pleased, so thankful to have you. And despite you saying that your support is given under a type of family duress, I still want to thank you, from the bottom of my heart – and if this is the last thing that comes from the bottom of 'MY' heart, well it would be worth it.

I Love you dearly John.

Max

End of letter

Day 22 – 21/04/10

It's been a nightmare today with my I.N.R level. Their path-lab's I.N.R reading is way lower than my machine, so they want to give me 3mg a day more Warfarin and Fragmin injections until my I.N.R goes above 3.0. Absolute nonsense. Been doing my I.N.R for five years and have been on 9/10/11mg the whole time, Freeman stick their nose in and now I'm on 12mg and 14,700ml Fragmin injection. It is all so pointless. They are overmedicating me, but it's 6 PM and no one is around to argue with. And I'm not certain enough to refuse to take their doses, so will have to wait and query it tomorrow.

Warfarin, I think, is managed extremely poorly in hospital and I don't want to get into having a blood test every day – my arms will be punctured more than an embroidery cloth! Still, I shouldn't get so annoyed about it really – when the transplant comes, my Warfarin will be discontinued!! That's a good point of transplant I suppose. So, just waiting around for my Fragmin injection, then will walk to Pam's, have dinner, watch some footy and then cruise back.

I don't know why I've got so frustrated at my Warfarin. I suppose because I've been doing it for so long so well, ultimately, I am offended when my management is discounted and overruled against my judgement. I suppose it is a sort of pride thing, which is silly really – considering they are giving me the kind of healthcare they believe to be right – but that's the way I feel. Also I am very conscious of having to hang around the hospital more for blood tests and nurse-administered medicine.

Hopefully they'll let me get my blood checked in the normal I.N.R clinic and continue to dose myself. I feel like saying that medicine is solely based on clinical evidence and the clinical evidence is that me and my machine are working fine – so you shouldn't be intervening.

Dr Hasan wants the main Haematology consultant to come to see me – he's the man in the know, apparently and he said he would get him to come and see me tomorrow to sort it all out. Dr Hasan is just so helpful. I saw him when I was walking out to go home and he asked if the blood consultant – Dr Castavan – had been to see me yet. I said no and he immediately got on his phone to sort it out.

Oh for some reason I do hope it's Dr Hasan that does my transplant. Massimo is very good also, but Dr Hasan is the main man!

I suppose I might have to wait around for most of the day tomorrow to see this Haematologist – still, makes me realise how rubbish it would be, up here, if I had to stay in all the time and therefore makes me appreciate the freedom they are affording me.

Spoke to Becky from work today and she has a cousin who lives in Gosforth – just down the road from the hospital and she is coming up to see her this weekend. Me and Pam are going to meet up with her and her cousin hopefully on the Saturday. She's so nice Becky – kept asking if there is anything I, or Pam, or Alex need that she can bring up. So nice.

*   *   *

You know sometimes I feel quite guilty. I feel a little ashamed of myself with some of my thoughts about my heart. I berate it in my mind sometimes, sometimes I swear at it – I even can, every now and again, feel repulsed by it – when I replay some of the words doctors have used to describe it … 'a big bag full of blood, not really doing anything' and 'ventricle like a balloon, blown up and up, with the heart wall stretching and thinning' and the worst one of all, 'it's like a ticking time bomb and no one knows when it will go off.'

I feel let down by my heart, disabled by my heart and even tormented by it. I used to think, when I had my aggressive palpitations, that my heart was almost teasing me, almost laughing at me, at how it is terrorising my life. I sort of thought of it as a kind of villain – a vindictive evil that dominates me sometimes – sometimes to the point when I would – although I only did this a few times – thump my chest to try to hurt it…Shameful. But that's what I've done sometimes, when I'm in a rapid atrial flutter, or on a really, really tired day.

I have created a monster in my mind and called it my heart – and I have attributed all of my faults, all of my fears, all of my personal insecurities and frailties to its make-up. I have created a terror and one which, most importantly – and here's the thing – I can hate and I can blame.

I have packed together every ill and limitation and problem I have, wrapped it in a black cloak, giving it a sunken, sallow face and staked it down to the beating muscle in my chest cavity. And this is why I now feel so guilty and ashamed – for at the end, I realise, I am wrong. Everything is not how it seemed.

I have written previously about how poorly my heart is and how unbelievable it is that I am so well. And really, when you think about it, this miraculous health and amazing quality of life is, all my heart's glory. Even though systolic function is measured at only 15%, it still fills me with life. Even though the right ventricle is massively volume loaded, it still fills with life. Even though my atrial rhythm disturbances further decrease efficiency and my valve lets blood go the wrong way, it still fills me with life. My heart has got me here today and has done so despite its problems and its bad luck. It has constantly worked tirelessly for me, when it could have given up long ago – but still, it beats on.

So, I suppose, now, at the end of our time together, I really need to say just two things – sorry and thank you. God Bless. I can't think of anything else to say, I just hope that when I move onto my new life, my old heart remains with me in virtue, if not in person.

Day 23 – 22/04/2010

Well, couldn't get to sleep last night. Turned the TV off just after 11, but they didn't turn the lights onto dim in the hallway, so my room remained just too bright for me to be able to get to sleep. Tossed and turned and then tried out my Alice band again, which worked so well for me in the Heart Hospital. But, now, when I put it over my eyes, it feels like it's pushing them too much and therefore is too uncomfortable to get to sleep.

When it got to near midnight I thought it was stupid that the corridor lights were still on full. I mean even if the night nursing shift was running behind – which it was – I still don't see why they can't put the lights onto dim – it's not like it's pitch darkness, not even close.

Anyway, in the end, I thought I'd push my nurses buzzer to ask them to turn the lights down. As I pushed my buzzer I could hear the nurses outside saying, '...that's max...', '...what? Max? Hold on...' and then a nurse appeared at my door within moments. Just think they were shocked and concerned, because in my three and a half weeks here, I haven't pushed my buzzer once. Bless them, they were so concerned. Even after the nurse left and dimmed the lights, I heard her talking to the other nurse, '... is he okay Emma?', '...Yeah he's fine, just wanted the lights off'. Ah they are all so nice here.

But, then with the room finally darkish, I just, all of a sudden, became really upset. I miss being with Pam. I just started really, really crying. I couldn't stop. I cried for five minutes, stopped for a little and caught my breath, thought that was the end of my outburst, but then burst out sobbing, all over again. This went on two, or three times. I was just so upset. Felt, in those moments, so sorry for myself. I just felt so, so sorry for myself – in this poxy hospital bed, agonisingly close, but worlds away from my wife – who is sleeping, alone also, just a few streets away. Kept thinking, *I don't want to be here – here in this room. I don't want to be in this bed – I want to be with Pam.*

Oh it's just so sad that I have not cuddled up with Pam to sleep for three and a half weeks and this is just the start. Could have months more waiting yet – and could be weeks and weeks after transplant also. It's just so sad. I so want to cuddle up to her, spoon her and find that nook we both fit into with each other. But I've got to be in this hospital bed. I've got to sleep by myself on Ward 30. I just cried my heart out for that sole reason – I felt so sorry for myself and could not stop the tears. It's just so horrible being pulled apart from the one you love, especially when geographical distance is not the reason.

Anyway, after a good quarter of an hour of weeping, my eyes dried and I did, then, fortunately, get asleep quite quickly.

* * *

You know my I.N.R mystery has intensified. I did a trio correlation test this morning; a finger-prick blood-drop on my Co-ag machine, then, from the same drop of blood also, on the hospitals Co-ag machine and another venous blood test. Results were: my Co-ag 5.4, Freeman's Co-ag 2.9 and venous blood sample 3.0. It would seem that my machine is well and truly knackered, however the head Haematologist consultant came to see me – an older man who clearly really knew his stuff – who, by the way of recompense, agreed with me, that prescribing me 14,700ml of Fragmin, was a bit of a waste of time. He also said, if I can write this without sounding too arrogant, that people who manage and are – long-term – responsible for their own I.N.R management, probably know more about it all than any S.H.O (Senior House Officer) – which makes me feel good, because it's easy to disagree with what the S.H.O's prescribe and to know that the top blood consultants, on the balance of things, would back my judgement, just makes me feel quite good. Sort of like restoring the confidence that I felt was being taken away without explanation.

Anyway, the consultant Haematologist wasn't as quick to condemn my machine, so tomorrow we are going to repeat the trio correlation test and if my machine is still that much out, then he will send it off to Roche Diagnostics to investigate further. And in the meantime he will give me one of their machines to use, so I can go on testing and dosing my own Warfarin! He said the last thing we want to do is take away your confidence in managing your Warfarin, especially when I have clearly been doing so well with it.

The other piece of news today is... guess what... it's to do with Alex... it's... oh it's so exciting... he's... he's... he's got another tooth cut through!!! Yay!!! On his right of the middle top teeth, one has just cut through. Ah bless him. He's so cute and he's just coming on leaps and bounds – sitting up by himself now for ages, rolling over, slapping away his bottle decisively when he wants no more, starting to look around for people – like when you're pushing him in his buggy and now he has his third tooth... yay. It's all just so amazing and wonderful. He's only a week off being eight months old. He is really, really thriving I tell you and I could not be more happy and proud of that fact.

That night I watched the Prime-Ministerial debate between Nick Clegg, David Cameron and Gordon Brown. Nick Clegg was sickly, pious and pompous. Gordon Brown seemed quite humble and simple and for once not telling you what your issue is and David Cameron was assured, but did at times, seem a bit scared. Strange isn't it, that so much of our vote on National Governance comes down to if someone looks calm, talks well and is assured of himself. You have a nation's infrastructure, economy, security and foreign policy in the hands of a selected cabinet and yet if the leader – who is not a security general, who is not an economist, who is not an engineer – appears, in any way, unappealing, then the control of the nation will not be given to them.

I think it's just a flaw in all of us. Let's face it, most people who vote would not know the Transport minister's name of the party they voted for – least of all the sort of person they are and what they'll do and how they will probably treat their position. Yet that lack of knowledge does not at all matter when it comes to 'the vote'. Why? I suppose because we do not want to bother with it. No one wants to be bombarded with details do they? Who wants to know specific bills that each parties want to pass? Who wants to obtain a full knowledge and understanding of each party's ministers and their beliefs, hopes and professional desires?

All people want to know is headline policy promises and of course what the leader of the party is like. Sure, the leader is important – his personality is important – but so is everything else – however no one really cares for that do they?

'Who you going to vote for?'

'Don't know, but I like Nick Clegg' – that's what it comes down too.

People may look for a few individual policies that are relevant to them, but that's it. The running of a nation decided on such little grounds. There's probably more fuller and wider ranging scrutiny given to a company employing a cleaning firm, than what the average person gives to their vote and party of choice. Unbiased evaluation of a political party, I do not think, occurs much.

But what the hell do I know? I suppose it's always been like this. As I said on day 1, liking, or not liking someone, is so important. I mean who's going to vote for a party in which they just simply do not like the leader? You can bang on about the unbelievably huge levels of media intrusion nowadays and the addition of these televised debates, making the election more of a personality contest; more of a PR advertisement as much as you like, but I suspect that long before these things, people still generally voted for who they liked, or, in the negative, would not vote for someone they didn't like.

It may well be that for a long, long time, the governance of this country – indeed any democratic nation – is decided by which leader shows the most endearing and likable personality. I only reckon this, because everyone gets to vote now, so the power to decide rests with the people who – perhaps only in times of relative wealth and ease – would rather read The Sun, or watch only one particular channel's news to gain all the knowledge they need to vote.

Now who's being pompous and arrogant – Nick Clegg eat your heart out!!!

I know I'm young, unlearned, not schooled in the history and theories of democracy and I only pay fleeting attention when I do get interested, so I'm probably way, way wrong. But it just seems to me that the decision as to who to vote for is so, so important, you can only do so if you've gained a full, unbiased, rounded knowledge of all three parties and their ministers and their record. And you can't get this from the newspapers and news channels. So you have to independently find out for yourself; on the Internet, in libraries, talking to various people who are more learned on it all.

But who can be bothered to do that? Certainly not me and I'm sure not the majority of voters. So, really, you could say that the bulk of us are just throwing darts in the dark, when we vote.

I have no idea who is best for the country, or who is best for me and my family, so it would be wrong for me to vote really. You wouldn't let me have a say in the peri-operative treatment of someone just out of cardiac surgery, because I have no knowledge. To a lesser, but still great enough extent, that is why I will not be voting – oh and also because I'm an inpatient, in Newcastle, awaiting a heart transplant.

And if I had to vote, I'd vote Conservative – why? Because Dad did and I don't like Gordon Brown. And that's all. Not good enough reasons, I feel, to be allowed a say in the matter.

But this has always, I think, been one of the problems with democracy. The joke in Blackadder, about being pleased the likes of Baldrick don't get a vote:

'...and a good thing too, give people the-likes-of Baldrick the vote and we'll all be back to wandering around like cavorting druids and dung for dinner.' So funny.

But democracy gets away with it, because the blame for the problems it causes are everyone's fault and that's what the world likes – at least the one we live in. Although you may be able to run a country better under other systems, ultimately, if the country goes down and becomes bad, no one person can be blamed, as we all have the government we deserve in a democracy. I mean a dictator could get more done, but not many would be able to cope with the responsibility of things going wrong and a country's blame being aimed squarely at you and you alone.

It's safe if it's a democracy, but, I do not think, necessarily fairer. For what is politics, other than trying to find a compromise between the nations irreconcilable wants, with a finite use of resource. Rather them than me.

'Or do you think that's just bollocks Les?' Ha-ha, just a private joke there from Men Behaving Badly. Anyway, that's enough politics I think for one day.

Day 24 – 23/04/2010

Had a really good night's sleep last night. Got asleep quite quickly and didn't have any nasty, bad dreams.

Had to wait around in room today because the I.N.R lady was going to come and see me and lend me a new machine. She came round at about one-ish. She was really nice. She had two, new-model, Co-ag-u-check S machines with her. One was their master machine, which is calibrated to their path lab and is completely accurate and the other was a spare from the cupboard.

She tested, simultaneously, her I.N.R on the master machine and the one she was going to give me and they both read 1.0 exactly. Perfect. Then I tested my blood, simultaneously, on her machine and my old Co-ag-u-check; my machine read 4.4 and her machine 2.9.

So looks like my machine is not accurate and, probably, for a long time, I've been running my real I.N.R far too low, which is supposed to be really dangerous for me. Oh well, just another lucky escape I've had, it seems.

So, now on 12 mg per day and will do everything the same except use the new machine. What's best about that, is that now I have a machine we all trust, there is no need for the S.H.O's, or paediatric registrars to stick their noses into my Warfarin management. So, after two, when Linda Robson, the I.N.R woman left, I walked to the chapel to have a little play on the piano and then went back to the house.

However, it was such a lovely day that me, Pam and Alex laid out over the park with handmade, Italian ice cream. Mmmnn, was well nice. We gave some ice cream to Alex. He loved it! Think it soothes his painfully-teething gums and also tasted really nice. He held the cone himself and ate lots of the ice cream and munched some of the cone too, without choking, so bonus there.

After that I had a nice bath at the house and Pam made a lovely roast pork dinner. Alex was grizzling a lot though, because of his teeth we think, so gave him some Calpol, although this seemed to appease very little.

*   *   *

It's now nearly 9 o'clock and I'm back in room writing in my journal, as you can probably guess by the existence of these handwritten words. Also, you can probably guess by the thinning of blue ink on the previous page and the abrupt change of colour to black, that another pen has been used up.

That's three pens I've used up now writing this journal. Ok, the Pilot G-1 pens I'm using do not have too much ink in them and, also, I use up a lot of ink doing things like... ~~ultatate~~... ~~don't you rekon~~...scribbling stuff out! But, even so, I can't believe how much I've written. What started as a time killer, or hobby, has become so, so much more. And I didn't plan on it being so. I just thought, *I know, I'll keep a journal, that will give me something to do and something to pass a bit of time with* – but it's become so, so much more.

I even think twice about leaving the journal in my room when I'm out; how crazy is that! Who's going to take something from my room, let alone a journal and this is a hospital, but that just shows you how much I treasure these pages – to the point of completely off-the-wall worry about losing them – it just shows you what it means to me.

Anyway, enough of that I suppose; writing about my journal,

in my journal, is a bit like a dog chasing its own tail, so I'll stop it now.

Well I suppose that's all for today then. I suppose I'll see what's on TV, but my hopes are not high! Get to see Becky from work tomorrow – don't tell Pam, but she is well hot...crap – Pam's well going to read that ... Sorry Pam!

Oh and she's bringing my work computer up too, so that's way cool.

Catch you tomorrow Journal – perhaps I should give you a proper name, instead of keep calling you by the common noun – but perhaps not. Oh Max, you've clearly run out of things to say – put the damn pen down...oh okay, but I just want to... NOW!!!

Ok, Ok. Night. –x-

Day 25 – 24/04/2010

Had a really, really good day today. Before I'd even blinked in the morning an S.H.O came round to take my blood and then, at about 9:30, Dr O'Sullivan and Massimo, came round on their morning rounds – in normal clothes, because of the weekend.

Dr O'Sullivan asked if I've been going out, so I said, 'yes.' But then he asked me how far I'd gone. I was going to lie and just say Jesmond, but thought I'd be honest and confess I'd been into Newcastle – I'm not sure if I'm really allowed that far – however, Dr O'Sullivan didn't bat an eyelid.

So, it was 9:30 AM and I had a Carte-Blanche for the rest of the day.

Cruised to the house and watched some snooker with John, then us four went over the park, which was packed, due to the glorious weather and had a picnic lunch.

Then, at just after 3 PM, we all went into Newcastle to meet Becky and her older cousin Sissie – strange name I know – at the Marks and Spencer Delicatessen Cafe. It was really nice. We stayed with them for a couple of hours; Becky, Sis and Pam shared a bottle of Chardonnay and I had a tea and John a coffee. They both adored Alex, who was giving them big smiles – who wouldn't adore him though?

Becky gave me my computer which – although I should now be able to get onto the Internet – I still can't use, because I can't remember my password! I had a few goes guessing, but then the computer said that I had tried to log-in too many times and shut itself down. When I rebooted the computer, it loaded this strange security checkpoint page, with a funny username and password prompt, which I've never seen before. I'll have to call I.T on Monday, but I just hope they can fix it over the phone, or I don't know what I'll do.

Pam and Sis switched numbers, because she only lives in Gosforth and is around in the day times and said to Pam that if she ever needs anything, or wants a place to go, or someone to go out with, to give her a call. Was so nice of her and she's really, really friendly and knows Newcastle really well for any advice.

We then cruised back home and had a lovely, home-made, fish pie for dinner. There was a bit of a disagreement as to whose fish pie it was – I made the cheese sauce, mashed the potatoes and sweated off the leaks and spinach, but Pam assembled it all and baked it in the oven. It would be common just to say that it was a combined effort, however Pam had this strange assertion in her mind, that I was her sous-chef! And therefore the Pie was her making.

Tish I say; everyone knows that the white sauce and mashed potato make a nice fish pie – considering neither of us have control over the quality of the fish – therefore, I should take most of the credit. However, John thanked Pam much more, so shows you where his allegiances lie – although, did you expect anything different?

*   *   *

It's now 10:20 PM and I'm back in my hospital room contemplating what next to do... watch TV – there are a few good films on I think – watch another 24 episode on the PSP, turn lights out for an early night – although the hallway lights are still on full, so doubt I'll get to sleep, or keep writing in the Journal of doom? Urmmn, I just don't know.

You know a thought has just struck me. Had a glance back through the previous pages and it seems, to me, that I haven't written about the actual transplant in days. Maybe I have a little, but certainly not to a significant degree. What does that tell you? That I've slipped back into the other world, where all this mortal talk of transplantation is again, just an illusion? A night stalker of bad dreams and altered reality? Does it mean that I am just in denial of the actual reality I'm in? Or could it just be, that I'm coping oh so well with it, that I haven't needed to torture myself about it constantly and therefore have not written about it in a while?

Well, most people will think it's the latter one, I reckon. And they are probably mostly right, but I do disagree with how well people think I'm coping with it all ...

Sure, I'm coping sufficiently and I have not yet fallen apart – but, until you fully understand what 'coping' actually is, implicitly, you can never really be sure. I know that coping is a product of the human spirit and therefore not subject to objective quantifying – so you could say that it is an exercise in futility, trying to evaluate how well I am coping with all this – like on a scale of 1 to 10 say.

But that is what you all want to know isn't it?

'How is Max doing?'

'How is he coping?'

Well, if I knew how to answer that I would, but I haven't got a clue, because ultimately, I have no idea what coping really is. And even if I had a rough idea of what it was, it would be, deep down, unique to me; so, when Mum and Pam and me have to answer that question we all say, 'he's doing really well. He's really upbeat and positive. He is really okay.'

And don't get me wrong, these are all true, but does it answer the question? I don't know. Do these facts – and they are facts – mean that I'm coping? Again, I do not know. I suspect I am coping, as most would agree, but how much and for how long? Who knows... or dares to dream.

Night –x-

Day 26 – 25/04/2010

Mummy is back up to see me... yay! She got to the house at noon and we went for a nice, slow, long walk around Paddy Freeman's and had a lovely roast chicken dinner, which Pam made. Also played Nomi and again Pam pipped me at the post to win – I just don't know how she does it. She seems to just sneak up on the outside to take victory, time and time again. But don't worry – I'll get her!

On the way back in the evening me and Mum saw Dr Hasan as we came in the main doors! I just always seem to bump into him. And even on a Sunday evening at 7:30 PM he is still here, slowly strolling around.

Had a really nice long talk to Lulu. She read me a pupil's letter to her school's Headmaster and we argued about politics and Louise called me obtuse; don't think that I have ever, in my adult life, had a discussion/argument with Louise without being called obtuse. However, no one else has ever really called me obtuse, which may be because all the other people I argue/have discussions with, would not use the word obtuse – because they simply either do not know what it means, or they are not comfortable enough with its meaning to use it – or, perhaps, because they do not think that I am obtuse.

And if the latter is the case then, Lulu, you have an issue with obtusity! Or maybe it's just because I'm her younger brother and Lulu is an English teacher, with a teacher's mentality when it comes to arguing! Oh but I absolutely love her to bits, just the way she is.

Anyway, we worked it out in the end and she finally saw my point and I hers... but I was still right! Don't tell her that though.

Tin Cup is on ITV3, which is just such a good film. I watched it sort of recently though, so I'm not too worried about watching it – I've just got it on in the background; don't tell Emma though – apparently she hates the TV being on in the background when you're not really watching it, because of the distraction it causes – a tendency she revealed when she was up visiting with Legsy, half drunk, in the Chinese.

Okay, so have just turned the TV off so I can pay more fuller attention to my writing. Let's see if Emma is right. Let's see if the first part of today's writing is, in comparison, less focused than this next part, due to the TV's distracting influence.

When will I have my heart transplant? The unanswerable question. The source of so much uncertainty. Just when will it be? When will the time come to pass? When will there be 'the' knock on the door, or 'the' phone call whilst I'm out wandering in the daytime. No-one knows do they?

And it's not like every day that passes you get closer to it, or it becomes more certain, or anything like that. I'm just waiting and then, all of a sudden, it will be time. There really is no middle ground is there?

I thought maybe coming here and being trapped in the hospital would be a sort of progression to the transplant, but it's not really. The waiting is the same here as it would be at home. But I'm not so sure that I'm actually waiting. I don't really think that I am waiting for a heart transplant you know...

Real waiting – for anything – can only occur when something is almost certain to happen, real soon. You can only wait – actively wait, as opposed to passively wait – for something, when that something is imminent and when your immediate surroundings are the surroundings in which the thing will be.

If I'm catching a bus tomorrow morning at 9 AM, when I go to bed tonight, you would hardly define that time as waiting for the bus ... would you? Once you get to the bus station the next morning you can say you're waiting for the bus.

I know this all sounds childishly obvious, but it's an absolutely critical distinction for me and the transplant wait. You see, by the factors that I've just described, I am very rarely waiting for a heart transplant. I am only at the bus stop when I am awake, in this room – and even then it doesn't much feel like I'm waiting for a bus, because not a single one has come by in nearly four weeks! So, really, I'm not really waiting.

I was when I first got here and I still do, sometimes, when I'm in my room and think, or have a feeling, that the bus to the anaesthetists room is approaching. But, just as quick as I think that, the feeling has gone – or the sound of the oncoming footsteps in the hallway, were the sound of a domestic's feet, or a doctor's feet for another cubicle... not me, not yet; still not a sign of a bus.

Logically, I know it will eventually come, but for now I'm either enjoying a different, but still lovely life away from hospital, or am just sitting at this seemingly deserted bus shelter.

The waiting, it seems, is as absent as that bus.

WEEK **5**

Day 27 – 26/04/2010

Before I begin, I must glue in a poem Mum wrote to me yesterday. She had read my bit about coping and wrote the below in the wake of that.

Mum's writing

> *He says he's not coping,*
> *But what does that mean?*
> *Does it mean he's not hoping?*
> *Or daring to dream?*
> *Does it mean that he is moping?*
> *And wanting to scream......*
> *That he's slopping and spiralling down on his knees.*
>
> *He says that he is coping,*
> *But what does that say?*
> *That he is welcoming the sunlight of each new day?*
> *That he is eating and sleeping and feeling just fine,*
> *And his life is just dandy until it comes to 'that time'.*
>
> *He wonders if he is coping,*
> *He is managing 'well',*
> *I'm his mother and I know – I know him very well*

End of Mum's poem

It's a lovely poem. All I would say is that the last line should be changed to, '... I know him <u>so</u> well' – just like the song; although I can't remember which song.

Also, whilst I'm in a logistical, practical mood, I will glue into the Journal the menus you get here at the Freeman for the hospital food. It is so, so nice and wanted a record of the choice and type of food you get here – it's all so nice.

The Newcastle upon Tyne Hospitals **NHS**
NHS Foundation Trust

Name _Crampton_

Ward _CRS_

Breakfast Menu

Please shade the black box next to your choice like this ■

☑	Chilled orange juice	HE
☐	Porridge or	HE
☐	Bran cereal or	HE
☐	Cornflakes or	HE
☐	Weetabix or	HE
☑	Rice krispies or	HE
☐	Muesli	HE
☐	Croissant or	
☑	Fresh banana or	HE
☐	Grapefruit segments or	HE
☐	Fruit yoghurt or	HE
☐	Wholemeal roll or	HE
☐	White bread or	HE
☐	Wholemeal bread	HE
☐	Butter or	
☐	Polyunsaturated margarine	HE
☐	Jam or	HE
☐	Marmalade	HE
☐	Sugar or	
☐	Granulated sweetener	HE

SMOKEFREE

Do you smoke and want to stop? You are **four times** more likely to quit with NHS help.
Please ask the nurse caring for you for information, **or** contact the free NHS help and advice telephone line:

NHS Free Smoking Helpline: 0800 169 0169

Diet code
HE = Choices recommended for healthy eating and diabetics

For Ward Use Only

☐ Assistance required

Lunch menu

The Newcastle upon Tyne Hospitals **NHS**
NHS Foundation Trust

Name CRAMPTON
Ward CBS
Monday Lunch 1

Please shade the black box next to your choice like this ■

☐	Chilled orange juice or	HE
☐	Home made cream of mushroom soup	HE
☐	Chicken & mushroom pie or	
	Select pieces of chicken with mushrooms in a white sauce topped with a puff pastry lid	
☐	Vegetable burger with ratatouille or	
	Vegetable burger served with onions, peppers, courgettes and aubergines bound in a tomato sauce	
☐	Hungarian goulash or	HE
	Locally produced beef steak bound in a tomato and paprika sauce with potato garnish	
☐	Egg salad or	HE
☐	Roast turkey & stuffing sandwich	HE
	Served in brown bread	
☐	Gravy	HE
☐	Salad cream portion	
☐	Creamed potatoes	HE
☐	Parsley potatoes	HE
☐	Cabbage	HE
☐	Butter beans	HE
☐	Syrup sponge &/ or	
	Lightly baked sponge capped with Golden Syrup	
☐	Custard sauce or	HE
☐	Cheese & biscuits or	
☐	Fresh apple or	HE
☐	Raspberry jelly	HE
☐		

— Would you like an afternoon snack? —

☐	Mini pack biscuits or	
☐	Individual cake	

For Ward Use Only
☐ Assistance required

SMOKEFREE

Do you smoke and want to stop?
You are **four times** more likely to quit with NHS help.
Please ask the nurse caring for you for information, **or**
contact the free NHS help and advice telephone line:

NHS Free Smoking Helpline: 0800 169 0169

Diet code
HE = Choices recommended for
healthy eating and diabetics

The Newcastle upon Tyne Hospitals **NHS**
NHS Foundation Trust

Name CRAMPTON
Ward CBS
Monday Evening 1

Please shade the black box next to your choice like this ■

☐	Chilled orange juice or	HE
☐	Home made scotch broth	HE
☐	Beef in mushroom sauce or	HE
	Beef steak served in a rich tomato and thyme sauce laced with onions, garlic and mushrooms	
☐	Macaroni cheese or	
	Macaroni in a light cheese sauce topped with Cheddar cheese and oven baked	
☐	Ham pizza or	
	Deep crust pizza topped with tomatoes, York ham and Cheddar cheese	
☐	Cottage cheese and pineapple salad or	HE
☐	Tuna, mayo & cucumber sandwich	
	Served in brown bread	
☐	Gravy	HE
☐	Salad cream portion	
☐	Creamed potatoes	HE
☐	Chipped potatoes	
☐	Peas	HE
☐	Sweetcorn	HE
☐	Semolina or	HE
	Semolina pudding with milk and sugar	
☐	Cheese & biscuits or	
☐	Mandarins in natural juice or	HE
☐	Ice cream	HE
☐		

— Would you like an evening snack? —

☐	Mini pack biscuits or	D
☐	Individual cake	

For Ward Use Only
☐ Assistance required

SMOKEFREE

Do you smoke and want to stop?
You are **four times** more likely to quit with NHS help.
Please ask the nurse caring for you for information, **or**
contact the free NHS help and advice telephone line:

NHS Free Smoking Helpline: 0800 169 0169

Diet code
HE = Choices recommended for
healthy eating and diabetics

And just for no reason, here's a trace of my hand.

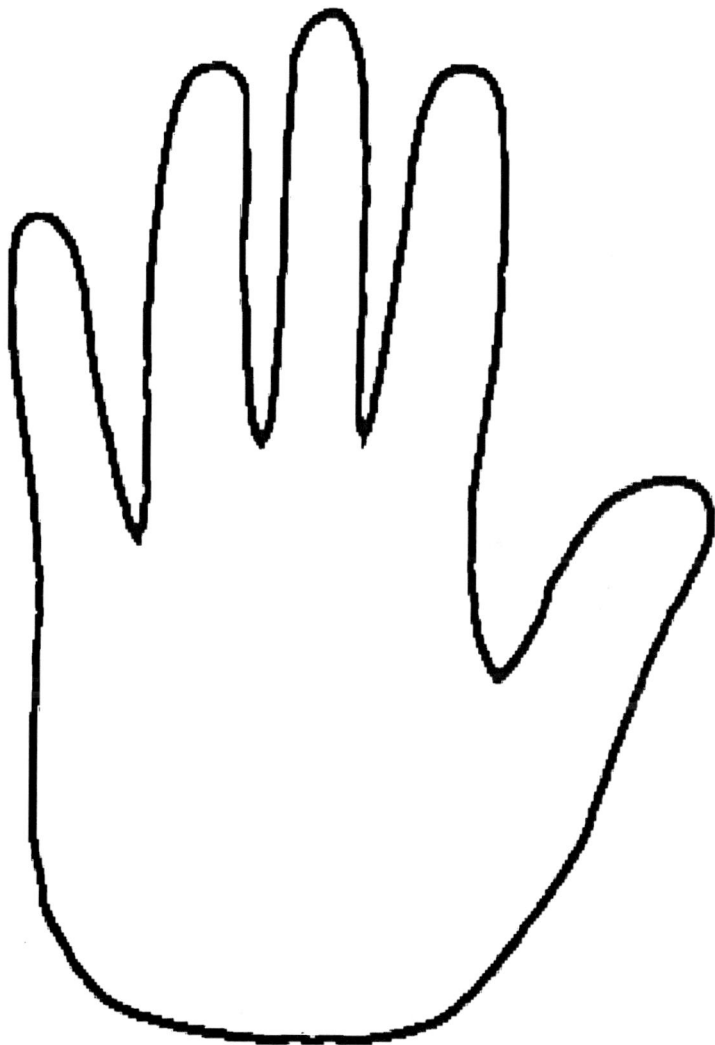

Now I know what you might be thinking... is this guy for real? Has he finally lost the plot? Lost his mind? Has he become an absolute mentalist? Have the stresses and strains of this situation, this life, finally broken him? Am I going insane? Well, sorry to disappoint, but I'm afraid I'm not; the truth is a whole lot plainer and pathetic.

You see the pages of this journal are running out. Only 12 left at the start of this day's writing. So, clearly I need to buy another one – as I have been doing with the pens I've been using.

I'm writing with a Pilot G-2 for all you stationary enthusiasts out there – a break from my more favoured Pilot G-1, but an interim that is by no means to my handwriting's detriment, I don't think. Although this Pilot G-2 was just meant to be a stopgap, a substitute, whilst I bought some more G-1s, I now think I will continue writing with this one, until it's empty, even though I have now replenished my G-1 stock with two, brand-spanking new, Pilot, gel ink, roller-ball, G-1, fine-tip pens. They will just have to wait their turn because the G-2 is in town.

Oh god I'm talking about rubbish. Still, I'm embarrassed to say that the subject I was going to write about, but went on a tangent from, is about as interesting as the tangent itself. So by judging the sheer insipidness of the G-1, G-2 talk, you may want to look away now – as they say on the news when revealing the football scores.

Anyway, back to my point! Come on Max, you can do it. Okay, as I was saying before, the life of this most trusted and dearest journal is coming to an end. And, like the pens before it, I need to have another one, before this runs out, so as to ensure that I'm never without quill, or parchment, even for just one evening – because when inspiration strikes, it doesn't wait around for losers without the means to act upon it. And I don't want to be one of those losers.

So today, when me and Mum were in town, I bought myself another journal to take over when this one runs out. However – and I feel bad writing this in this journal (please forgive me journal) – but the new one I bought is just well rock and roll. It's genuine tan leather, with parchment shaded pages and an elastic clasp to keep it closed. It just well looks the business.

Apparently, when Pam bought this journal (which is still well cool), the one that I've just bought was only available with lined pages – no thanks! No self-respecting journal writer would buy a journal with lined pages – the ignominy of it! But, this time in WH Smith's, the nice tan-leather journal was available in plain, sepia pages, so I wasted no time in snapping it up.

However, now, as I like the look and feel of the new journal so much, I really want to get to the end of this one, so that I can legitimately start the other one. I know I could forgo these last pages and just go straight into the new journal, but that wouldn't be fair to this journal – and this journal definitely deserves justice for what it has become and I could not bear to finish it under disingenuous, or corrupt circumstances. The new journal may be a Rolls-Royce, but this Ford Fiesta has got me this far, so it's right and proper, to give it its just-desserts and pen it to the end.

However, this nobility, or strict moral stance, does not go as far as to what has to go into these last pages – cue the menus and very random hand trace. To be brutally honest, I've done them so I could get to the end quicker and thus onto the new journal. Ok, ok – I know I've just talked very high and mightily about respect-fully giving this journal its just-desserts and that filling these pages with menus and handprints is little less than outright cheating, but I am no saint and my moral integrity only stretches so far; it is not total and therefore my line is drawn, before just jumping straight into the new journal, but after some quick, space consuming, meaningless, page fillers, such as menus and handprints. There. I hope you all place me somewhere to the right middle of a savage-to-saint ethical scale!

I can't believe it, that four pages have been taken up by glued in prints, hand traces and stationary talk. I can't believe it. When reading back this will be a real low point in the journal's interest, me thinks. Oh well, you can't be profound, deep, or interesting all the time can you – I mean just ask Pam!!! Boom-boom . . . only joking! :-)

Well, I suppose I should tell you what I got up to today, instead
of just boring you with pen, journal and glue-in talk. Well, I had
such a nice day. Spent virtually all of it exclusively with Mum.
Mum, Pam and Alex came over to me at about nine, then Pam
and Alex went off whilst we waited for the doctors. Alex fell
asleep on my bed drinking his bottle – oh he is just so cute! An
absolute darling.

No doctors came round, just Debbie and Amanda and at the
same time Kirsty came up to introduce me to the new transplant coordinator – I've forgotten her name already – but Mum
had popped out to get a coffee and when she came back she
saw me standing in the corridor with all four nurses and her
heart sank, because she thought that this was going to be it!
But she soon realised it wasn't when she saw the four of us
joking about. They were taking the micky out of my dress
sense, because I had on pyjama shorts, socks pulled up and my
Crocs. Debbie said that just because I'm up north, doesn't
mean I can let my standards slip! They are quite funny and
really, really nice. Amanda told us about the shuttle bus from
Central Station to the Quayside, which is meant to be really
good – perhaps we'll check that out.

Anyway me and Mum then went to the chapel to play the
piano – I played her Tom's song, 'I'm Wondering Why?' Which
she hasn't heard before, then we drove into Newcastle for a
little look around and some lunch.

We went to Frankie and Benny's which was nice, however,
Mum sort of choked – throat closed up with a rogue catch of
Balsamic vinegar – and she really was in distress for a few
seconds. She said she tried to breathe about 2 to 3 times and
her throat just remained closed. She went red and stood up
with fright. She was going to run out of the restaurant, but after
a big gulp of water, it seemed to clear. Was quite scary though
and must have been terrifying for her. How awful going to
breathe and your throat just being completely blocked!

Anyway, after we avoided the death throes of Frankie and

Benny's, we did a bit of shopping; Mum bought some flip-flops
... ooo, whilst I'm in a silly mood, I just can't resist noting down
my relevant joke:

*'What do you call a Frenchman in sandals.......? Philippe
Flop!'*

Haha – but back to what I was saying ... Mum bought some
flip-flops and I bought my extremely over described, aforementioned journal.

Then we cruised back to the house – I hit snoozy city for a
little bit (crap, Mum has just told me that 'little' is spelt with
one 't', but think for my whole life I've been writing it with two
'ts', so will take some getting used to the correct spelling) and
then we all played Nomi again and again – yep, you've guessed
it... Pam won!

I am just completely miffed as to how she keeps doing it. I
don't think she is cunning enough to be able to cheat to victory
and... hold on ... oh crap... I just remembered ... John won,
not Pam! Well that thought has cheered me up a litle (yay, spelt
it right!) Yeah, I remember now, because John called 'four' on
the double-blind hand and absolutely nailed it, securing him a
cool 60 points – a massive single hand score and one which,
considering he was already leading the pack, put him out over
the horizon in terms of catching him for victory. I gave it a good
go though and it did, in the end, come down to the last hand,
however, I was never going to win. I had to call 'three' on the
three-card round and win all the tricks – a task hard enough to
do, even with a good hand, let alone the crap one which I was
dealt on the last round! Still, was a really good game.

Then me and Mum went to the Indian next to the lovely
Chinese for dinner. Well, well, well nice – one of the nicest
Indians I have had I reckon – it was gorgeous. We had
Popadoms, Peshwari Naan, Onion Rice, Spinach Bhaji, Lamb
Rogan-Josh, a Garlic and Spinach Chicken dish and a side order

of plain Vegetable Curry. I know it sounds a lot, hell, for two people it is quite a bit really, but we pretty much finished the whole lot, save for a few spoonfuls of Spinach Bhaji, Vegetable Curry and some Rogan Josh sauce. Mmmmnnn, I do love my food you know.

Mum came back to my room for a litle then walked back to the house.

Stop the presses. . . . . . hold the phones. . . . . . it has just come to my attention that, as I thought, 'little' is spelt with two 'ts'! I thought it sounded really, really strange when Mum said that. It's only because I consider myself a terrible speller, as I'm sure you can see when you read this journal, that I didn't have sufficient confidence to argue back at Mum and tell her to stop poking her nose into my 'little' spelling! And now I've written a whole paragraph a page back saying how I've got to get used to spelling it with one 't', I've made myself look very foolish.

Still, this didn't perturb Mum in still finding and highlighting, other spelling mistakes, even after the 'little' clanger! I wrote somewhere earlier that I was '. . .a little board. . .' – accidentaly spelling [in the original text] the word I wanted, 'bored' as the wooden plank 'board'. I mean clearly I know the difference, just in my haste I wrote phonetically, instead of thinking about the correct spelling, but Mum pointed it out, thinking that I didn't actually know the difference.

I said of course I know how to spell 'bored' and more to the point, in that sentence in question, at least I spelt 'little' correctly! Haha – got her there!!

Well, couldn't sleep in the night. Was going to switch the light back on and start writing again. Turned lights out at about 10:30 and was wide awake at midnight when there was a lot of commotion outside – lots of alarms and running feet in the corridor. The arrest trolley – which is just outside my door – by no more than a coincidence, I hope, was scrambled away down the corridor, so think someone was in trouble and crashing. Not that this woke me up – I was still wide awake before and after.

Night-time in hospital is becoming – it seems by the last few nights – quite hard, lonely and uncomfortable. Still, I'm hoping all I need is a few good night's sleep to dispel such slowly encroaching ills. Let's hope aye. I have had a few bad nights here, but the last two have been particularly hard, with ever longer tossing and turning and mental unease – and they have been on consecutive nights, which always makes the situation worse. Still I refuse to worry about it. I probably fell asleep in the end around 1 AM, I suppose.

But what's nice now is that the nursing staff do not wake me in the morning to do my obs, so I slept in till around 8 AM. Mmmmn, nice lay-in, yes please.

Day 28 – 27/04/2010

When Debbie and Amanda came round this morning, they said that they had an offer on a heart last night for me, but Great Ormond Street, in their words, nicked it. Close one aye – I could nearly have had it done last night man!

Had lovely day. Mum and John walked Alex into Newcastle and back again after we had lunch in the house. This meant that me and Pam had a good few hours together for ourselves, which was really, really nice. We just went straight upstairs, to bed, to snuggle and snooze together; we wasted not a second finding each other's nook – burrowing down to that warm and soft, buttery feeling of each other's body, gripped tightly within our arms. We stayed there for about two hours. Drifted in and out of sleep. It was lovely. Another moment I could have happily let last forever...

You know I've written it seems, so much about the dangers of my heart, about the risks of transplantation, about the fear of the whole thing, about the pain of changing worlds and about the terror of my own mortality. But, I don't think I've really noted down what a transplant could, or indeed would, do for me...

Being born with Ebstein's anomaly is not a good thing. That much is obvious I suppose. For all my life, I have not been able to do certain things. Throughout my life there are pleasures and joys that I have not been able to experience. For all my life there have been simple, basic activities, I have never been able to do ...

To run. The most basic and natural freedom you can have – fight or flight is hardwired into our very make-up and yet I have no flight. It probably is the single most overriding limitation that I could announce. For there are many disadvantages leading from my disability to run:

Football, run-outs, tag, first one to the shop wins, legging it when playing bud-ups, or knock-up-ginger, P.E at School, Fun Run day; although no one liked this and it was one of those rare times when the Ebsteins was seen as an advantage, because I could get out of it! Foot races with friends, Bulldog, batting at cricket, quick cricket, rugby; although again, am not sure if it was the Ebsteins that kept me from rugby, or just my better sense of good judgement. Well that's just a few of the limitations of not being able to run, at any point, during my life.

Another problem with Ebsteins is stamina. I have very, very little. And this affects so, so much:

Walking up the stairs when the lift or escalators are broken, walking up steep hills not being sure if I can make the top, sometimes, just walking around a theme park and being too tired to carry my own weight. Washing my car – I have to stop very often to build my strength back. Screwing in a large, hard turning screw – I can only manage one and that's with rests in-between.

There are just so many painfully simple things that I (although can still do), massively struggle with and am never certain, at the outset of each thing, whether it is something I can do, or not... like:

Putting up a flat-pack wardrobe, getting the weekly shopping in from the car in one go, walking to work on a knackered morning, holding little Alex in my arms for a while, carrying my backpack whilst travelling, painting, hoovering, any kind of housework – honestly, I'm not just writing that as an excuse, I honestly would rather be able to clean the bathroom and then go and clean the windows, without having to sit down and rest... honestly.

Playing more than a couple of table tennis games consecutively, walking up the hill back from Woodbridge to the cottage, kneading dough to make bread, changing a light socket above my head; arms soon become leaden by the burden of their own weight, being sucked down by gravity. Cutting the grass, sweeping the decking, wheeling a heavy wheelbarrow, pushing Alex in his buggy, keeping up with friends' pace when walking home from school and if I couldn't keep up, pretending to kneel down to tie my shoes, as a ploy to buy some rest time. Climbing ropes in gymnastics, being on my feet all day on school field trips to Calais. Sometimes, on a really tired day, which Ebsteins can easily deal you, I've slouched and hunched over, just standing in the shower; the effort to support my own weight just so, so hard to bear.

That's the lack of stamina and strength. But there are other limitations I have only discovered as I have grown older – indeed the older I get, the more limitations I realise I have. It's horrible. It's like the older I become, the more I realise has been taken away from me, like:

When buying my first property there were certain mortgages I couldn't get, because they required life insurance, which was too expensive and not available to me. When going out to get my first job, I was struck by the amount of jobs that I couldn't do – anything that wasn't an office job really. When going out to night-clubs with mates, I would get so tired on the dance floor – trying to dance without actually achieving it, to be honest – that I would want to leave early and go back sooner than my more energetic friends. When travelling I couldn't Bungee jump, or skydive, due to the G-force pressures my anti-coagulated body would be subjected too. Also, depending on which country I went to, depended how much travel insurance would cost – an expense much greater for me. Surfing was too knackering, most walks through South Africa I couldn't even attempt, because of the hills and distance – even day trips could be too physically demanding, depending on what they entailed. Diving with wild dolphins – although I could do, I had to come out of the water much quicker, because the current was so strong and fighting against it too great a struggle for me, so had to come back to the boat real quick. Deep sea diving – I haven't got the puff for and am not allowed – white water rafting, cycling, horseback riding on the beach, even paint-balling are all, really, out of my reach.

And there is another ominous grouping of new things I would not be able to do, but have not yet discovered; being a father and the millions of things I wont be able to do with Alex, or do for Alex are slowly going to come to fruition.

I have only written four pages on my physical limitations – I could easily have doubled, trebled, or even quadrupled that – honestly. And that's just the physical effect. Mentally Ebsteins has scourged me too.

I always say I have Ebsteins anomaly of the heart and of the head. The impact it has on you when you simply cannot 'rely' on yourself, physically, is just as hard. When not being able to get asleep really worries you, because you know you won't just be tired the next day, you will be super-tired. When embarking on a long journey and worrying about just not having the strength to walk to the baggage reclaim, or walk up the stairs to passport control, after a long flight. The thought that any cold, or fever, or ill, will affect you much, much more than normal. Just the state of mind, I suppose, to sum it up, of 'doubt', is rife within my perception of anything physical to do with me – and this omnipresent doubting is no more than the mental scar of Ebsteins.

Now, I want to go back to my first few sentences about all of this... 'for all my life, I have not been able to do certain things. Throughout my life there are pleasures and joys that I have not been able to experience.' Well – and this is what I have not mentioned so much yet – a successful heart transplant will, to the repeated sentences above, enable me to add the same two words onto the end of each of them; perhaps the most important and meaningful two words I have ever added to a sentence... the two words are, '...so far.'

And when you re-read those two sentences, with those two words added on the end, you realise – well I do – the seemingly infinite possibilities, joys and pleasures of a heart transplant. For only in my wildest dreams may such a reality lie... 'what dreams may come...' -x-

Mum made her legendary Toad-in-the-Hole that night, which Pam, for some reason, calls Sausage-Toad! Madness. Then we had another game of Nomi and, for the first time, Mum won!! She was as surprised as us, I think. The overriding factor was the double-blind, double-points hand; Mum wildly guessed five tricks and absolutely nailed it – giving her an eye-watering 70 point haul. Unbelievable – have never seen anything like it. Of course this shot her into the lead at such a distance there was no chance really of catching her. She did play really well though.

Mum then walked me back to my room and I did get a really nice night's sleep.

Day 29 – 28/04/2010

Not sure how much I've kept you up to speed on my work-computer fiasco. Last I think I wrote was that I locked the computer and had to call I.T. Well, as it is a laptop and is therefore away from the safety of the office, it is installed with a sort of decryption and if you enter your password wrong too many times, it not only locks you out of your user account, but also paralyses the computer, until the special decryption password gets re-entered. However, I.T Security keep this password a closely guarded secret and therefore, despite my unusual situation, they cannot tell me it over the phone.

So, to cut a painfully long story short – which should never have been this long to begin with – Mum is taking my computer back down to London today, so I.T can unlock it, reset my password and then it can be couriered back up to me, maybe as early as tomorrow. However, I bet the courier this time is not as hot as the last one... (again, sorry Pam).

So, Mummy went back about midday. I have so enjoyed spending all this time with her. It really, really flew by; it really did. I tell you, honestly, it's such enjoyable, relaxing, quality, quality time spent with one another, that when I think about it, the memories are more in line with a lovely holiday, or special weekend break, rather than an actual hospital visit. Isn't it just mad.

It seems at the moment, the more things progress, the more paradoxical they become; a healthy stable man who is critically ill, awaiting life-threatening surgery at any moment, but feels more relaxed than ever. Being dragged away from my home, family, friends and life which I love, only to find equal love-of-life in Newcastle – a place that has been forced upon me. And things like this recent time with Mum, just make it starker; Mum just been to see her son, in hospital, awaiting a heart transplant on the transplant list, but coming back with the feeling of being on a wonderful vacation, or much-needed weekend break.

It all just makes no sense to me, no sense at all. Where is the pain...? Oh I've tempted fate now – Max you idiot!! But it just astounds me how extraordinary and deceiving and surprising and downright unbelievable life really can be. I had such a lovely time with Mum though, I truly did. Was sad to see her go, but not too sad surprisingly, I know I'll see her again soon and I talk to her every day, which I really like.

Watched Avatar after Mum left and had a bath with Alex! He has been in the best mood all day. He has been laughing so much at seemingly everything and anything. He looked a little unsure at first about getting in the bath with me, but he soon took to it. We had to cut it short though, because I.T called about my new password, so had to pass Alex to Pam to take the call.

Pam then cooked a lovely Spaghetti Bolognaise for dinner, although as usual she laid the plate with 17 tonnes of Spaghetti, which is a pet hate of mine; too much pasta dilutes the sauce, which is, quite obviously, the best part! Anyway, I shouldn't be too harsh, as it was really nice and I polished it all off, except the excess pasta.

John walked me be back to the hospital amidst the most warmest and pleasant evenings we've had here weather-wise. The air was still and the evening light soft and plain. Everything seemed to have a slowness, a calmness about it; from the old boys playing bowls on the bowling lawn, to the easy, relaxed pace of mine and John's footsteps. Everything seemed gentle, sure, soft. It was a lovely evening to walk back in. And I got a good night's sleep to-boot.

Well that's the end of day 29 and of this first journal, but still barely the start of this whole thing called Heart Transplantation.

- x -

God bless and goodnight – see you on day 30 in the new journal...

Journal Two

Day 30 – 29/04/2010

A new journal, but still the same old heart. 30 days I've been writing, but still no transplant. I have, we have however, still done much, in this first month; rented a wonderful three-bedroom house, moved Alex and all our stuff up to Newcastle and John and his stuff too. Found our way around the Freeman Hospital, High-Heaton and Newcastle town centre. Become friendly with lots of staff: Asif (Dr Hasan), Lynne, Kirsty, Amanda, Debbie, Milind (DR Choudhury), Hannah, Helen, Linda, Tessa, Dr O'Sullivan and Mark – plus a good few more I don't know the names of. I found and played the piano, worked out a type of day-release with the paediatric team and even got John sorted with his I.N.R testing in the clinic here.

In short, we have settled into things up here in such a way that, so far – and it's important, not just negative, to say, 'so far' – that we are not thinking, or longing for our lives back down south yet.

Really we are just fine here and are in no way mourning the loss of our normal lives – we're just content with this one up here, for the time being. And I suppose, other than actual transplantation, this is the biggest and best thing we could have done, so far up here, in these first 30 days.

I suppose that we couldn't have used them better, or hoped for them to have gone any better – again other than a successful heart transplantation procedure!

And this being the case, I'm so proud of me and Pam and these first 30 days. We have both done so well. Also John and Mum – our two pillars of strength and support – have passed everything with flying colours so far and have created the environment for mine and Pam's strength to breed and grow and make this time here, what we have made of it, so far.

We are doing really well. I guess that's all so far I can, or need to say. You should be oh so proud of yourself Max; you really should.

Had pretty much a routine day today. Pam and Alex met me at the hospital, then we cruised back to the house. We then walked to Sainsbury's and later I had a bath and won at Nomi when we played it – nearly broke my Nomi point scoring record of 270, but just missed out with a total end score of 265!

Nothing else to mention really about today. We saw Kirsty kicking around the hospital and she said that the G.O.S.H teenager is now off the transplant list and also someone who was my size and blood-group in Harefield has also now been transplanted, so I am right up the list now I think, although I'm not exactly sure of the transplant list's rules, or indeed if there are any – think it may be a first-come-first-served basis, so it's good that two people ahead of me have now been done. I really do think that the transplant will be at any moment now; here's wishing...... or dreading!

Day 31 – 30/04/2010

Had quite a good night's sleep I suppose. I was quite wide awake when I turned the TV off at about 10:30-ish, however I was comfortable and didn't toss and turn too much.

Bobby text me a few times as he was meant to get a call on Wednesday from the team here to see if he is allowed onto the heart transplant list. However Wednesday and yesterday (Thursday) he didn't get a call, so he is calling in today to chase them up. He said in his text message he hadn't heard from them and that he's going to phone in today, because he can't go the whole weekend without knowing.

So, so much uncertainty, all of the time. It is just so hard for all of us. I'm in no way alone in my struggle – and although I know that logically, to have it directly shown to me, on my mobile phone, just brings it home I suppose. Hope he finds out today, but with hospitals, you just never know.

Guess what? Pam has just called me to tell me that my computer's just been delivered. How quick was that; it was only couriered yesterday morning. So Pam is bringing it over now – excellent aye. Oh crap, downside is that now it's 'back to work!' Only joking, that will be good for me – it really will.

Anyway I probably got to sleep at about midnight, maybe after, but slept soundly.

So am just sitting in my room awaiting doctors, Pam with my laptop and my liberty for the day. Not sure what we'll do today? Go to Newcastle? Go into Gosforth? Go to the theatre, or be taken into theatre? Who knows? I'll see what Pam, John and the Gods say...

Well, I waited in until 11 AM for the doctors, but no one came, so went to the house. Weather was absolutely glorious; shorts and T-shirt weather! So me and John, well admittedly, it was much more John, cut the grass in the back garden. It looked like the previous tenants had never cut the grass, as it was so overgrown; it took the pair of us hours to do it.

Was lovely though; me, John and Alex were all in the garden – Alex was sitting in his pushchair in the shade, chatting away to us and kept pulling off his sun hat – and Pam spent a good few hours in the kitchen making Alex another lovely bunch of food up. She did a cod and tomato pasta dish and this well-nice smelling Nectarine, Apple and Strawberry thing. Alex eats like a king I tell you – which is no less than he deserves.

So us three were busy working and Alex was getting some lovely fresh air whilst on-looking. Was such a domesticated afternoon, it really was – other than it being a Friday and not a Sunday, it really could have been, literally, an afternoon from my old life... me cutting the grass whilst Pam sorts out Alex's food and us keep having breaks to play, or chat to Alex. In that afternoon High-Heaton has never seemed so similar to Little-Thurrock; it was really nice.

Well I suppose I've got to write about what happened when we played Nomi that night. I really don't want to, but before you can move on from something, talking about it, is the first step. And for me to heal from what happened, I must write about it – as a way, I suppose, of exorcising the demon, that came about, on tonight's fated game of Nominations!

Well, I came last, but that's the least of it. Pam won and she, with seemingly no effort at all, broke the legendary 300 point bracket. It was quite something. She finished on 300 points dead and – and this is the part that pains me so – gloated like there was no tomorrow. The 300 points is put into more perspective when you learn that she was down on the double-blind hand, so she could even have had much, much more.

But the gloating... I've never seen anything like it. Every hand she was up on, she stood up and done a silly dance – which, as the game progressed, turned into a silly, taunting dance, solely around me, with her ducking her head down to my left ear, then right ear, to exclaim a certain note in a stupid, stupid tune, that she was humming, to accompany her dance. And as her points went up, so did the absurdity of her gloating repertoire. Soon she was dancing around the whole table, humming a cheesy, whining type tune, turning round to wiggle her bum at me and then prancing off again, back around the table.

At the end she wrote all over the score-sheet proclaiming herself the 'Ultimate Champion' and crossed my name out and replaced it with the 'Ultimate Chump'. But believe me the gloating didn't even stop there.

After the game, Pam dropped me back at the hospital and carried on that damned annoying victory tune all the way. Also, when leaning down in the passenger seat to replace the parking permit that had fallen down, I banged my head, quite loudly, on the door frame. Of course this set Pam off in hysterics; she then started to incorporate the Nomi win and head injury incident, into the lyrics of whatever song was playing on the radio. Let's just say I slammed the radio off – but this didn't deter Pam.

Now you may have thought that after Pam had dropped me off, the gloating extraordinaire would have ceased – I mean it was only a Nomination victory, however I was wrong. When I got back to my room, over the course of about an hour, I received a picture text from her, John, Louise, Liza [Tom's wife] and Mum and the picture was the same in all five text messages… it was the end total of Pam's score from the score-sheet – the photo was of a scrap of paper below;

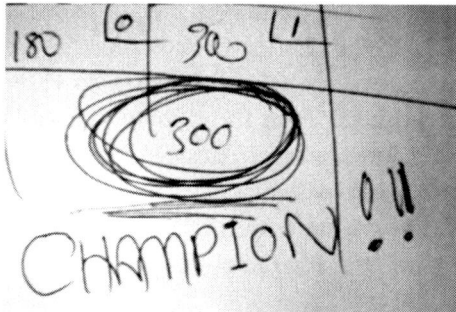

I tell you that girl does make me laugh. What gets me though, is that all this gloating is aimed at me! You would have thought that I usually win Nomi and therefore any gloating should be aimed at me, but I hardly ever win. John and Pam have probably won twice the amount of times that I have! It's just so unfair!!!

It was really funny though – I mean if you can't laugh what can you do? 'Take up politics perhaps' (Blackadder). But I tell you, I've never seen anyone, so overexcited and gloating over a single game of Nominations – never! Needless to say that it took me a while to get asleep, but wasn't too bad.

I briefly spoke to Mum; when I called her she thought it was going to be it… 'the' call. You see she's convinced it will happen on a Friday – my cardiac arrest was on a Friday, as well as the time I was called up here for the false alarm and also when they put me on the list and told us about staying in the hospital – that was a Friday too. So will it be tonight???

Day 32 – 01/05/2010

No. That's the answer to yesterday's closing question. No. No action, no call, no transplantation. Hey-ho, never mind, am sure it will be soon though.

I got my computer working completely properly yesterday. I overcame three separate problems and got it working myself, without having to call I.T. I was well proud of myself. First I overcome an Internet parameter problem when trying to connect to the web – I renewed my I.P address and then it started working. Then I had a 'proxy-nomadis' error, so I tried switching my target server from London to Paris Head-Office and then that worked. Then the dongle stopped working and came up with a funny error. Thought I was stumped, until I realised that the software disc was still in the disc-drive and therefore was interfering with the dongle, so I removed it and everything is now working ticket-ee-boo. Bravo!

So it's Saturday and am just waiting in my room for anyone to come and see me. Guess what? Back out of the window, for the first time in a good few weeks… grey soup! It's as drab as a constantly rented, but never refurbished, 1970s, council flat. And it's quite cold too. Have just put my jumper on, which is a garment I haven't used in a while. Because of the crappy weather, I fancy going into Newcastle today. But we'll see what the others want.

Well I'm not sure now what else to write about. I really don't know. I don't know how much journal I'm going to be able to write after my transplant, not sure how I'm going to be doing, but I'll try as hard as I can – but don't want to get into the habit of writing in the journal, for the purpose of just writing in the journal… oh crap, that's what I've just done… Oh Max… Sort it out.

Yay, Dr Choudhury has just come to see me, so I can go now. Woo-hoo… catch you later on today … or tomorrow … or in I.C.U…

* * *

It's 8 PM and I feel crap. I feel completely fed up and down and am in a right pig-of-a-mood. I don't really know why. It is a miracle that I am even writing about it, such is my state of abject indifference and complete dejection. I feel utterly depressed, annoyed and slightly angry – although anger is an emotion that requires will and I have such little bother for anything right now, that I do not even have the mental resource to be properly angry; it's more like an echo of anger, a reverberation – which in some ways is even more infuriating, because you know that not even your anger has enough breath to survive, for any real amount of time.

And I suppose that is the overriding, fundamental part of complete and utter dejection – that no feelings are decisive enough to hold on to; with no volition to do, or think, or want for anything either. It is a total and coherent shutdown of any will, or impetus, any hope, joy, or even fear – for that matter. It's like a state of blankness, like a mood of absolute indefiniteness.

Being this fed up is rubbish. Complete crap. Can't be bothered to watch TV, go on the Internet, talk on the phone – hell, it is a testament to this journal's pull that I am even writing about it. You can stuff Newcastle – its wonderful doctors and lovely nurses – stuff it all. To hell with the poxy-bloody-infuriatingly-intolerable transplant! It is repulsing me even to write that word. Sod it all.

This stupid hospital and pointless, worthless ordeal. I'd throw it all in the bin, in a blink-of-an-eye, without so much as a nostalgic look back at it all.

The endless, endless talk. The endless, endless writing – which I'm bloody perpetuating right now. The endless, endless worrying and planning and surmising and contemplating and guessing and preparing and accepting and conversing and dissecting and analysing and hoping and justifying and tolerating and fighting and coping and bearing and thinking......

endless, endless, endless thinking – just all go away! *GO AWAY NOW*! Just go away – all of you – all of it. Go! GO…..! Just leave me alone.

Ultimately, when these moods strike and you feel nothing except aversion and condemnation towards everything and anything, you just want it all to go away and cease – for what's the point in all of it anyway? What's the worth? It's all stupid – the lot of it …

Sorry, you've caught me at a bad time – let's hope tomorrow morning brings more than just visual light. I love you all dearly – you all know that don't you? And by the pulse in my veins and beat of my heart it will always be so… long after these words and this journal have faded into time. Night –x-

Day 33 – 02/05/2010

Last night, after writing about my state of dejectedness, I read it out to Pam with a depressing, lifeless voice; in-keeping with the frame of mind I was in. She told me she loved me and we said goodnight. Then, less than 10 minutes later, Pam came walking into my room – it was just gone 9 PM.

She came to simply give me a cuddle and lay with me for a short while. I tell you my face lit up like a child at Christmas when I saw her come in. It was like a dream come over me – a splashing of warm scented liquid, rushing all over me; filling my cracks and holes within a flash.

It was a moment of such liberation, such saviour, that I find it hard to recount without my eyes watering. And Pam has done this exact same thing before …

A few years back, for no particular reason, all my friends were meeting in the evening, after work, to play football, down the ball-court. And obviously I couldn't go. Well actually I could and did, but I couldn't play – as my Ebsteins dictates. Anyway, for no extra reason other than that same sense of exclusion, I was really, really down and depressed about it, at work; the afternoon before the game.

Pam, who works only a few streets away, called about what train I was getting home and I, not knowing due to an unimportant problem at work, replied back to her saying that I didn't know what train I was getting and that I have got to work late; I also hung up on bad terms.

Then, at about six o'clock, I left the office and saw Pam in the foyer, reading her book, waiting for me. I couldn't believe it. Not only was I horrible to her on the phone – I didn't know when I was finishing, so she had no idea how long she would have needed to have waited for me. But this didn't bother her. She knew I was feeling really down, so she wanted to wait and go home with me, despite how long she had to wait. And what got me is that she didn't tell me that's what she was going to do. She just sat there, for only half an hour in the end, but she didn't know how long it was going to be, and just happily read her book.

I tell you that occasion and yesterday night are all I need to tell you, to show you how wonderful that girl is. Both times, last night and a few years ago, she helped me, she supported me, she rescued me in a way I've never known before. You see she was there for me, literally, physically, unquestionably, without mention, without announcement and without acclaim.

These two deeds are absolutely priceless and meaningful beyond compare, because they were so simple, so plain and just so perfect. It didn't take marching bands, valiant efforts, extraordinary endeavours, or end-of-the-earth sacrifice to show me her love and care and kindness. It was the fact that both occasions – well, maybe the first one more than last night – but both occasions were so unremarkable, so seemingly insignificant that they could easily have been passed over without thought, without action. But Pam could see. She could see what no one else could – that despite the commonness of both occasions, she knew she needed to take action and help.

It is easy for a lover to push a partner out of the way of an oncoming car – everyone would be proud to do that. But it takes someone really, really special to see the same car coming, in the guise of any day's quiet battle. I suppose what I'm trying to say is that most partners would be by their loved one's bedside in I.C.U, or rush home from work to be with them when a member of their family dies. But, I tell you, I reckon there are precious few that would be in the foyer of their partner's work, when they really, really need them.

And both times I didn't even need to ask. I didn't know I needed her, in that moment, but Pam seemed to know … she knew when I needed her – which is a rare bond that we have that really is quite something you know.

I love her with everything that I own and possess which is capable of loving. . .

WEEK **6**

Day 34 – 03/05/2010

Mum's writing

1:00 AM Max phones to say they have a donor. I am thrilled – he also sounds thrilled. Funny, he said it would happen before Tuesday and so this being Monday, he was right. He so often is.

I can't write this in order. At the moment it's 10 PM and my darling son (you Max) are doing so well. I can hardly believe how much progress you have and are making. You went down to theatre at 6:30 AM (apparently, you got through five razor-blades removing your body and face hair). At 10:30 AM your new heart was inserted and at 2:10 PM you were taken to I.C.U.

We spoke to Dr Hasan. He told us how well it went and said how good the heart was. He was smiling from ear to ear – I love that man!

Watching Pam with you, Max, is such a delight. She immediately goes to you – not put off by any of the paraphernalia – and strokes and kisses your face and brow, whilst uttering such gentle words of praise and love and care. Me? I was happy, more than happy, to just observe. I tell you that girl adores the absolute bones and sinew and fibre of you.

When you opened your eyes, it was the sweetest, bestest present ever. You even winked at me. And smiled. Well, half smiled because of the breathing tube. You sign-languaged: '*Yay, I woke up*' and then '*time?*' Then you got cocky and sign-languaged, '*when will I be extubated?*' Then you signed: '*ventilator*' – '*rock-on*' – '*I always hot*'...

Day 35 – 04/05/10

Pam's writings

Yeah besides others... a heart transplant didn't stop you from remembering my [Nomi] victory! You sign-languaged '*300*' and then '*screw you*'! It made us crack up Max.

YOU ARE JUST SO AMAZING.

Could kill these pages writing that over and over again. Here you are – mere hours after a HEART TRANSPLANT – all sedated, recovering from having your heart taken out (can't believe it's true... still seems like something from a science-fiction movie) and a new one put in, with tubes and drains coming out of you everywhere I look... bandages concealing the wounds from your heart transplant and I.C.D removal... and you are entertaining us!
  You are fine, you are safe, you are here,
  You are mine, you are Maxwell.
  My Darling Maxwell... and nothing, not even a heart transplant can stop, or change that. I love you so much!!!
  All of the time we were waiting for you to go down to theatre and then the actual wait whilst you were in surgery just seemed so surreal. To be honest I don't think I could really take in the enormity of it. I was so calm the whole time. Numb, I think is the best word to describe how I felt. I wasn't scared, apprehensive, nervous, tearful, or anything really... other than hungry. I could have eaten my weight again, given the chance. All I wanted to do was lay down quietly and eat.

In that sense the wait really wasn't that bad for me. I was more scared during your Electro-Physiology study, Ablation and I.C.D procedure last year. Bizarre aye?

Have to just interrupt what I'm writing to tell you that Alex has another tooth – the little darling. The big centre, top-right tooth, has come through in the night. And June has just spotted it. He's such a treasure Max. Don't think I'd have been so calm if it wasn't for him. He's such a tonic, such a pleasure to watch grow and develop. You two are my world. I love you both so dearly and completely. Anyway back to you. . .

So you called me at about 1:30 AM on the 03/05/2010. I was already awake listening to Alex stir in his sleep and you told me the words I have been waiting for, for the last 33 days ... 'It's time honey – they think they have a donor'. I pulled on my clothes, woke dad to tell him the news and drove straight round to you.

And this is where my awe and utter amazement of you began. . . you were calm and smiling sitting on your bed. We spent the next five hours together getting ready for your surgery – the X-ray, shower and disastrous shaving of your beard, chest and groin, phoning your family to say your 'see you laters' until after surgery. . . and your quiet calm never left you! You made it so easy for me Max. I couldn't have beared it if you'd been distressed and outwardly terrified, or if you started saying that you didn't want the transplant. I would have wanted to scoop you up and protect you and run away from the whole thing.

But you were brilliant! And your faith and unwavering peace and calm were justified. Here you are, the day after surgery and I am getting ready to come to see you at 10 AM and you are fine. . . the operation is over ... 'your heart is excellent' – Dr Hasan's words and the whole operation was perfect, textbook. . . as well as could be hoped and Asif couldn't stop beaming from ear to ear at delivering the news to us. He is such an amazing man Max and he so cared about making you well and giving you the longevity of life you deserve.

I went home after I left you in the theatre and scooped Alex up, cuddled him for ages, then fed him, changed him and before I knew it an hour and a half had passed... so much nicer than sitting in the waiting room.

At 8:30 AM, two hours after I first left you, Neil [Transplant Co-ordinator] finally called me to say you were finally under anaesthetic... I just thought he'd forgotten about me it took so long. He said they were going to start the operation and remove your heart, all ready for when the donor heart arrived at about 10:30 AM.

Your Mum then turned up with Dave and I filled them in on everything that had passed, before having a nice bath and relaxing.

At 10:20 AM Neil called again to say the new heart had arrived and you were all prep'd, ready to receive it.

At 11:30 AM he rang to say they were plumbing in the new heart and everything was going really well and you were lovely and pink, tolerating the surgery well. He said you should be done by about 2 PM.

By 1:30 PM your Mum, bless her, was getting anxious at no further updates, so we walked round to the hospital and sat in the waiting room and it was at about 2:30 PM that we saw Asif walk past. I jumped out of my chair and called out to him and he told us 'your heart is excellent and surgery went well.' He then said he was going to see how you were doing in I.C.U (all of this with the biggest smile you can imagine) – still in his scrubs from operating on you – my husband... amazing – couldn't stop smiling myself. He said we'd be able to see you shortly. Me and your Mum couldn't contain our excitement, she was crying tears of joy and me... well I just couldn't wait to see you and touch you again.

One of your nurses, Tracy, come to collect us from the waiting room about 10 minutes later and, bless her, she warned us that seeing you may be distressing due to all the tubes and wires. I thanked her for the consideration – but she needn't have worried. You looked absolutely beautiful to me, laying there all tucked up in bed with only your head exposed. They said you could probably hear me, so I smothered you in kisses, stroking your hair and told you, time and time again, that the operation had gone really well and you have a beautifully strong heart, how proud I was of you and how much I love you.

Then, about an hour later, you rewarded me in the best way possible by snapping open your eyes and looking at me for a split second, despite your sedation still being just as high a dose as when we first arrived. Oh it was amazing. Over the next half hour you continued to open your eyes occasionally and nod and shake your head to questions.

By 5 PM you were sign-languaging and making us laugh and smile fixedly at your speedy recovery from surgery. We were both so excited and relieved at how well the operation had clearly gone.

As you can probably tell I'm getting really tired now and my writing is getting smaller and scruffier. But just to finish. . .

We left you at about 6:30 PM to get some rest and the best present of the day came at 8 PM when I rang I.C.U to see how you were getting on and they told me they had removed your breathing tube and that I could come back and talk to you, even though it was outside visiting hours; 2 to 4 and 6 to 8. I hurried over and spent the next hour and a half answering all of your questions about the day:

- What did we get up to during your Op?
- What did Dr Hasan say when we saw him?
- How do you look?
- What did I think when I first saw you?
- The times of everything during the day?

The time just flew by. . . I massaged your feet. . . kept telling you 'no' when you tried to get me to sneak you extra water when the nurse wasn't looking. You were so, so, so thirsty bless ya!

You must have asked me every 5 to 10 minutes if you could have a bit more water, such was your thirst, but due to the anaesthetic you had to be limited to reduce the chance of you being sick and hurting your chest. The nurse just found you really cheeky and kept smiling at you. She was really nice and called Ivy.

Then I left you at 9:30 PM to enjoy a well earned night's rest, which, coincidentally, I'm just about to go and enjoy myself, as it's 9 PM on the 04/05 as I write this last sentence and I'm shattered.

Love you my baby!!

Sweet dreams and I will see tomorrow and pass back this journal for you to continue your masterpiece.

It's been a pleasure writing this for you and I hope I haven't missed too much out

-x-x-x-x-x-x-x-x-x-x-x-x-

Day 36 – 05/05/2010

Mum's writing

Took a photo of you last night.

That I cannot see you until 2 PM today is really hard. Perhaps we were spoiled yesterday seeing you in the morning for an hour, then another two and another two and now the long gap from 8 PM last night to. . .

Text from Sister Louise

> *Hold his hand for me Mum,*
> *Kiss his forehead for me Mum,*
> *Rub his feet for me Mum,*
> *Finger his hair for me Mum,*

Tell him I love him for me Mum -
So very, very, very much x

Just one of so many text messages. You are loved and cherished utterly by your family. You are highly thought of by so many and you are valued and respected by all who know you.

Max. This is your strength. Please take comfort and strength in everyone's love. Surround yourself with it. You were meant to be here. Take it moment by moment Max. Can't wait to see you. Here, so glad I got that picture last night! Love you dearly x

John says you look great

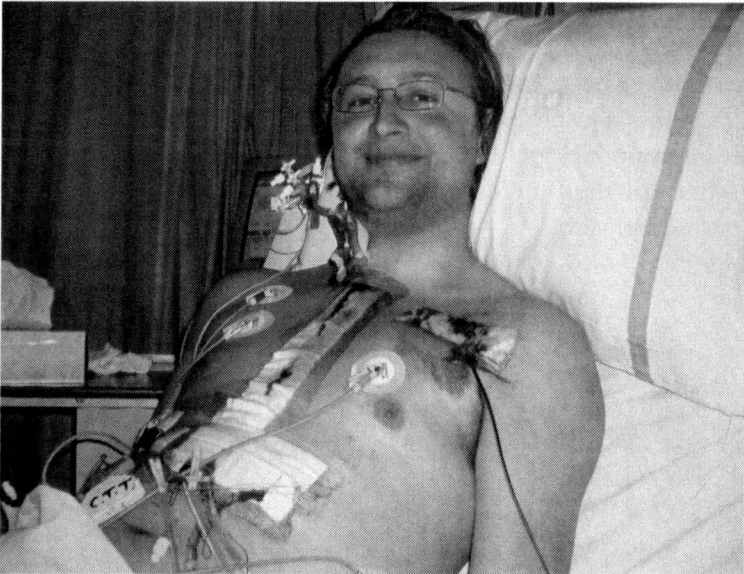

Day 3 Post Transplant – 05/05/2010

Me writing again

I'm in ward 27A. In an isolation cubicle for 7 days minimum. Not allowed out due to strong immuno-suppressant medication just started. This is too much. It shouldn't be allowed. But the only people who know that, it's too late for them. Oh what am I saying. It is awful.

It feels like a Joker has come over and sickly sliced up everything of pain and torture and blood and needles and suffering and rubbed them into my eyes, and pushed them down my throat, and laughed whilst doing it. This Max that is writing now is different. Oh so different from the one before – because I've been scarred by this here.

When I close my eyes I see blood – I see bulging veins, yellow iodine stained chest drains. I'm not seeing Alex, or Pam. Not in my mind. I've been possessed. Possessed by the corporeal essence of heart transplantation.

Oh this is just the blood and guts talking – you'll see. I'll soon come round. Hopefully...

Just coughed up lots more blood ... nice. This is all just so putrid and vile.

[Example of my handwriting on 5th May]

Day 5 Post Transplant – 07/05/2010

Didn't write yesterday at all and hardly anything for these other eventful days since Sunday. I will do my best to catch up. But I'll start from the present, 8 AM on Day 5 post transplant, the 07/05/2010 – Also Emma's wedding day today – and work backwards.

Last night I was really worried. Nurse said my blood-pressure was too high and that she had to let the doctor know. Then the doctor said she wasn't too sure whether to give me something, or leave it, so she phoned the consultant. Then the nurse came in with a tablet. Then, a few hours later, my blood-pressure was checked, but I didn't ask if it was okay; was scared bad news was going to start raining down on me ... heart not working properly ... rejection ... something else wrong which could be dire...

You see it's all been going so well, so far, that there must be some dangerous news, or big set back, or a problem with something somewhere...

Ah the doctors are outside now, all of them, discussing me ... Oh I hope it's good news. Am shaky whilst they're out there, it's so scary.

Anyway, let's change the subject. I have just had breakfast; Bacon, Eggs, Tomatoes (high protein diet), then Rice Crispies and a Banana, Orange juice and cuppa ... Mmmmnn, well nice.

Yesterday was better than the day before; definitely. Yesterday I had two chest drains out – only 3 more to go. I'm only on one Inotropic I.V (which supports the heart) and that's on a low setting. Also my pacing wires, that ensure the new heart rate doesn't drop below 100, haven't needed to be used yet, which is good; heart is beating quick enough with its own rhythm and Inotropic I.V.

Oh, doc's just come round and I'm not allowed my main chest drains out today, oh man! He said that because my heart cavity was so, so big, the new heart has lots of space around it, so the drains will have more to drain than usual and therefore they need to be left in more! Bummer! Still, I was allowed out my small I.C.D drain, which was cool. So another day with my drains in – I remember this from G.O.S.H actually; wanting my chest drains out and asking everyday! Patience Max, patience.

Boy I am so scared at the moment. My blood-pressure,

rejection, complications, kidney problems, the biopsy coming-up Monday. So much to be scared of. I feel okay – just really, really tired now – can barely keep my eyes open – but I'm on so much medicine now, I don't know if what I'm feeling is my feelings, or medicine-induced feelings. I am feeling pretty rubbish to be honest. I am so insanely tired right now and it's only 9.30 AM! Boy is this just well hard, or what?! Am still well tired.

Have spoken to Emma and Dan a good few times and they are having a really good day, although they said that they are well missing me and Pam and Alex.

My blood-pressure is still well too high. I don't know why I'm stressing about it so much. I mean it's not like high blood-pressure is a disaster, but it's the only thing that's not going right, so I am starting to worry … Is the high blood-pressure due to rejection? Will the high blood-pressure be able to be treated? Just so scared of something going wrong with this new heart and that being 'it' for me. But perhaps I'm just having a down moment … a scary mood. I mean I've just had my heart transplanted and have been on all sorts of medications and have been healing, which increases blood-pressure, so they just need to keep an eye on it and keep it down with meds, so just don't know why I'm stressing so, so much. I suppose I just feel really bad at the moment.

My back aches, head is fuzzy and compressed, body is weighted and awkward – I just don't feel really well at all.

Well the good news is that I've had another chest drain out, so I've only got one left now and also I'm fully weaned off all I.V medications – for now of course. So have just got pacing wires, E.C.G wires and left-lung chest drain now and can, independently, mobilise to the toilet; which I just did. And because my kidney function is good and urine output is good, they do not need to measure my in/out fluids – so I went a wee in the toilet … yay!!!

I can barely keep my eyes open and my mouth and throat is

awful; grainy and as dry as ash and my voice has pretty much gone. My chest is really clear which is good and haven't developed a temperature yet, so that's really good too, but body and mouth feel dreadful.

Pam should get here shortly.

Oh why am I worrying about my blood-pressure so much. Think my head is caving in and ears ringing because of blood-pressure symptoms – ridiculous; am just making things up now.

Ahhhh, have just put my fan on and am nice and chilled now.

Ooo just done a really deep cough and some puss oozed out of my main scar. I have a bandage on it, so it's getting it all, but the big cough made some dribble down the side where is was coming away.

Ooo am feeling a little more clear headed now – nurse just come around with a blood-pressure tablet. Perhaps that helped, perhaps it's just my mind.

Oh man where is Pam?

I mobilised quite a bit today; I stood up and marched on the spot and around my room for about an hour, which was really good. You know I'm really doing remarkably well you know. And the nurse, Tracy, just eased my worries about my blood-pressure – she said it's really common for blood-pressure to shoot up and down and that it's nothing to worry about. So that's cool. Also she can't give me my anti-rejection drugs, because my blood work hasn't come back from the lab yet – a problem with sending them this morning apparently. So I'll get them later. They are so on-the-ball here and to top it off Tracey, the nurse, is just making me a cup of tea!!! Rock on!

Day 6 – 08/05/2010

Had the best nights sleep so far. Wasn't disturbed, had no bad dreams, and awoke in perfect peace. Of course this was shattered when the realisation dawned on me of where I was and what my body felt like.

I got up to go a toilet and felt awful, became light-headed and heavy – not sure if from a deep, deep sleep I jumped up too quickly, leaving my new heart behind – or if it's just a physical aspect of my post-operative condition. Anyway, I made it back to bed unscathed except my ears were 'goldfish bowly'. And I am now sitting up writing.

My blood-pressure is still high, 167/87, but Tracy said they would adjust any meds for that. Also there is a third anti-rejection drug I should be on, except it's the one that's hard on the kidneys and my kidneys, apparently, are still not ready for a battering from them.

Have just read through Mum and Pam's writing again. Well what to write aye? All that waiting, all that thinking, all that build up; from first point of 'transplant' mention in April 2009 to now, May 2010 ... and the waiting is over. The Moment, finally came.

Just like the opening page, it was nothing more than the thundering rumble of inevitability. So what was that moment like?

I laid in the operating room, staring at the surgical lights, then Tim, the anaesthetist, said, here goes the first one (a little injection which makes your muscles sort-of-like freeze) and then, within seconds, I saw the next, main anaesthetic vial, pass over my head in his hand and disappear down to my cannula. I knew this was it...

So in my mind I pictured me and Pam and Alex, all cuddling into one another. That was the last thing I remembered ...

Then memories become distant, abstract, and highly questionable. I think the very first thing I remember is seeing Pam out of my right eye – left eye I think was obscured by the ventilator. Then just behind her I saw Mum. I then put my hand up to my face to see my pink fingers. In those seconds I knew I had survived – survived well, because I was pink and had normal visual/motor functions – no brain damage!!

I was thrilled. I started my sign language – and was pretty good at it too. Was surprised how much I had come around whilst still having the ventilator in, as the more 'with it' you are, the more they look to remove it. Anyway, think they were surprised how 'with it' I was with my current level of sedation . . . But I had my life and wife and Mum to look at, still there, me still with them; anaesthesia couldn't take that back away from me.

Time then is all quite hazy. Having the ventilator out, although lovely, is nasty. You just have to cough your guts up whilst they pull two tubes, wound all the way down into each lung, out. They gave me a suction tube to spit all the crap into and it felt like an entire throat and lung full of blood and mucus stuff; all up my nose, back of my throat and in my mouth . . . I just coughed and spluttered for ages, sucking away all that nastiness.

Then Pam was back, but I was super tired, so she just spoke to me for a bit whilst I closed my eyes.

That night passed like a blur, the next day pretty much did too. One well freaky thing happened though.

I can feel my new heart constantly pounding around my chest (they deliberately make the new heart beat really hard and fast) however, the beating sensation seemed to be in different places at different times – I figured it was just the way I was laying, or leaning, or something. However, when Mum and Pam were with me, I sat up and my heartbeat went to my throat!! It was actually my throat beating really hard! I shouted for help, or a doctor. A few doctors came over, but didn't seemed worried or even that bothered by my distress. They said my E.C.G was still fine and stable and saturations were good; they just thought I could feel some slight palpitations.

After say about a minute, my heart stopped beating in my throat and I was back to normal. However, when Dr Hasan came around, I told him about it and he said it's perfectly normal. He said I've had a sternotomy, which means my heart is no longer fixed into place – and also my heart cavity is much bigger than the heart they put back in, so my heart will, literally, move around and I'll be able to feel it beating in different places. He said the worst thing you can do is think about it.

Anyway, my only full day in I.C.U kind of breezed past and again time is a wholly different concept when in I.C.U. That night I took a Zopiclone sleeping tablet and I was out for the count.

Well, that sort of brings me to where I rejoined writing on Day 3, post transplant. I cannot tell you the psychological effects of I.C.U and the whole thing. My mind, for about a good day, was just possessed by wicked, evil thoughts. Awful, awful stuff which swam freely in and out of my mind; the drugs do it to you. For about a day/day-and-a-half, I wasn't me at all . . .

Nothing was reality. I didn't know who I was, what was happening, or where, or when, or anything . . . it was awful. The worst moments ever . . . the worst day ever. Am so pleased I managed to write about it, because that was what it was like for me, for a few days. Absolutely awful.

Oh, but I did get to see my new heart on the echo machine. I saw both ventricles, together, on the echo screen; [roughly drawn by hand. . .]

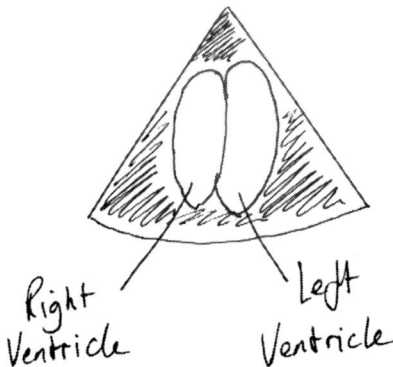

My echo used to be able to just show part of the R.V [right ventricle] on one screen;

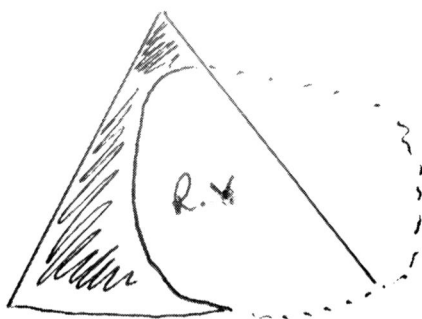

My heart was twice as big; the right side squashing the left so much and even inhibiting my lungs – I just can't believe how well I was with it – but, I suppose, the ultimate point is that I wasn't well with it; I'm now 'weller' without it. But, again, as I said in the other journal, it will remain with me in virtue. . .

WEEK **7**

Day 8 – 10/05/2010

Well, I've missed a few days. Writing in a journal everyday after a heart transplant is too hard. And writing about the ups and downs, highs and lows, pain, suffering and torture, of the past two days in detail, will also be too much, for there is simply too much of it all going on, to account for.

Yesterday and the night before I couldn't stand up; as soon as I did my head caved in and my ears rang really loud and I had to pretty much collapse onto the bed. Went from walking around, feeling great, to bed bound, in a day and I felt so down. Turns out I was extremely dehydrated and when I stood up my blood-pressure plummeted. Felt so scared; like something was seriously wrong. I was in a state.

And yesterday morning I had my first biopsy which was horrible as well. Especially as I was feeling just so, so bad . . . the pits. . . the utter, utter pits.

Boy, 7 days locked in this single room has been so hard. So, so hard. Pam has been here whenever I've needed her – she is so lovely. We have been snuggling on my bed at night for an hour or so; dreamy . . .

Day 9 – 11/05/2010

Well, I'm going to ditch writing about days, because they are all merging into one. So, just going to write in general terms with no order or chronology.

The last few days have been so hard. My body feels completely foreign; I'm a stranger in myself. My head is terrible. It feels like I've got 4 large, linen bed-sheets, squeezed through my ears into the back and sides of my head; it's so heavy and stiff and foggy. And my ears! They constantly hum, or ring, or kind of like reverberate – constantly in the background. The hum pervades every thought, or feeling, or turn... I just long for silence.

My neck feels like it's made of wicker baskets; it creaks and cracks at every movement and is stiffer than an iron rod. My hands shake, ever-so-slightly; as you can probably tell by the state of my hand-writing – and no jokes about my hand-writing always being this bad!

The left and right base underside of my tongue has been completely corrupted – it poisons everything I eat, or drink, turning it into a metallically, iron-like taste. Everything I eat is a chore, something I have to bear. I haven't enjoyed anything I've eaten since transplant. Also my mouth is just constantly dry; like my saliva glands are producing sand, instead of spit. My lips are dry too. My whole mouth is just a mess – and I so did love my food. I almost dread lunchtime, or dinnertime, because I have to almost force myself to eat. It's so sad.

My central line in my neck constantly irritates. It tugs and pulls at my side when I move and the I.V taps get caught on my t-shirt. And that's staying in for a while yet.

My room faces back towards the hospital, so there is no direct sunlight at all coming through the window. The room is always dark, depressing, lifeless. And the constant hum of the extractor continues.

A few days ago I completely lost my voice. It really was hell.

That couldn't be anymore crueller. I couldn't talk. I couldn't release anything – I was trapped, so much more than just physically. It only lasted about a day though.

I've just been started on two more horrible tablets: Magnesium and Calcium. Magnesium needs dissolving in liquid and then drinking; it tastes vile. I have to do that 3 times a day! And the Calcium tablet you have to chew once a day. They shouldn't be long term meds, but they could be.

It's really hard to go a wee. I have to really, really strain just to get a trickle – apparently it can be the effect of the catheter. That is annoying as well.

Oh it's just so long since I've taken pleasure from something. So long since I've really enjoyed something. At the moment everything is doom and gloom. Everything is grey and black, joyless and hard, struggle and effort, fight and bearability. I can hold on to so little good at the moment. I am just so, so down.

Everything is so hard and there is no let up … no peace … no silence – the hum in my ears still persists. At the moment, it's not so much that I can't see the light at the end of the tunnel, it's that I can't even look up to see it…

Day 10 – 12/05/2010

As you can see from yesterday, my worst times are in the morning. And I was really, really down yesterday. My head was at its foggiest and I was just so, so low. Cried loads to Mum. Cried to Pam. Cried when reading the above out to Emma on the phone.

But the day steadily improved. Went for a couple of walks around the hospital [*on the 11/05 my biopsy result was clear, therefore I was allowed out of my room*] and in the afternoon, the physio came up to do the exercise bike with me on the ward. That was well cool. Although I peddled with no resistance, the bike on the ward is a lot harder than the one in the gym [*shortly after my negative biopsy result came back the Physio came around and took me to the rehabilitation gym for a short exercise session*], so I actually got out-of-breath for the first time and it felt really good.

I rose my de-nerved heart from its rest-rate of 85, to 110 by the end of it. Now the 10 minutes on the bike was not that 'Eureka' moment, when I could do something more than I ever could before – I could still have done the 10 minutes with my old heart and maybe felt the same, or maybe a little more out-of-breath – however, there was other evidence of my new heart's ability.

When I got to the end of the 10 minutes and was a little out of breath, my SATs were 98%-ish still! Can you believe that? When I was out of breath slightly with my old heart my SATs would have dropped to under 90%. Doing just a walking test at my transplant assessment I walked, at normal pace, for 10 minutes and my SATs dropped to under 85%. I wont explain what SATs are, but just know that the less your SATs drop, the greater your exercise capacity is and therefore the better your heart is.

So, my rest SATs were 98% and after 10 minutes of exercise, my SATs were still 98% – meaning it took nothing out of me. Of course I felt tired in my legs and a little out-of-breath, but it is only 10/11 days after surgery. Well, it was well cool.

Then, later, we went for another walk outside and went to the Chapel to play the piano again – I went there in the morning, but was feeling so groggy, I couldn't play. But this time I played a few songs. Felt strange because my hands are a little trembly and arms a little achey, however, I did really enjoy it.

My head really started to clear which was so nice. In the evening, I felt really relaxed and comfortable, which was in stark contrast to the morning.

Day 11 – 13/05/2010

It's happened again. When I get up I instantly get light headed and head starts to pound. I have to sit down before I faint. As soon as I'm laying back down the light headedness goes, but I get this terrible ringing in my ears – really, really loud. Then my head just throbs. Great! Back to being an invalid again.

Was really worried, however, mouth was even drier than normal, so drank and drank and drank: 3 bottles of water, tea, orange juice and then, 20 minutes later, was completely back to normal. How mad is that?

In the morning my laying down blood-pressure was 180/90 (high, but they are medicating that – it's due to the anti-rejection drug side-effects) and when I stood up my blood-pressure dropped to 70/40! That's pass out territory. It dropped so low, so quickly that I even had to sit back down before the blood-pressure machine had finished it's measurement.

Last time that happened I was really dehydrated, so I drank all what I just mentioned and, literally, 20 minutes later, I could stand up like normal – no problems. How mad that 3 bottles of water can take you from a bed-bound, head-crushing, world-falling-in wreck, to just completely normal.

The docs are looking into the postural blood-pressure drop and my hypertension when laying down, but they told me not to worry and that I'm doing really, really well. Anyway, after the morning hiccup I was back to normal, feeling quite alright and my head still isn't that foggy!

Then I had, I think, that Eureka moment. Rather than going into detail, which I would usually, I will summarise what happened with a text I sent to family and friends. Well, the Eureka moment was at the gym session;

My Text to All

*In gym I just done more than I have ever done in 27 years.
That awful feeling of leaden-limbs, pulling me down, was still
there – I wasn't free from that like I thought – but, at that
burning point when before I just had to stop, today I just
endured it. The fatigue felt the same with the exception that
today I could still keep going. What dreams may come...*

Officially I did 10 minutes on the bike at level 2 – keeping it
at 80 r.p.m and then 2 ½ minutes on the cross-trainer, 40 step
up and downs, 20 squats, 20 heel raises, 30 thigh pushes on the
weight machine and 20 leg raises again on the weight machine.
Was well out-of-breath, fatigued and sweating, but felt just so
alive. I felt like I was really working out; properly, for the first
time ever! Was in gym say 30 minutes 'doing' the whole time.
    After I sent that text out I got the most wonderful response
from Louise;

Louise's Text

*Ah Max, you made me shiver. You will love it. When I swim
now I've built up such strength in my arms and body, the
water works with me and not against, and I feel so
empowered; effortlessly slicing up and down the pool and
never once feeling tired. There's no feeling quite like it –
STRENGTH. And you will, at last, know what that's like.*

Just reading that out loud to Mum made me well up again...

Day 12 – 14/05/2010

Well yesterday was certainly a good day. After gym they told me
and Mum that we were being turfed out of Ward 27A because they
needed the bed for someone sicker. Sounds like good news in a
way, however I'm being plugged into a 6-bed bay, on Ward 25; no
personal room, shower, free T.V, or D.V.D and what's worst of all is
it's back to normal visiting hours of 2-4 and 6-8.

How unbelievably pants is that! So annoyed. And what's
worse is that I had to vacate my room around 2 PM and my new
bed wasn't ready until 7.30 PM! So for all these hours me and
Mum just kicked our heels in the canteen, the chapel and Ward
27A's kitchen. Was a bit of a sham really.

But when I got into the bay I was next to the huge windows
that look out away from the hospital . . . finally natural sunlight.

As I got to my bed I could see the sun setting amongst the
trees across the way. It felt well nice.

Drank loads that night because of dehydration. Was up three
times weeing, but felt completely normal; not light-headed at
all – so that's cool. My head is feeling so much clearer too and
my hum in the ears is no way near as bad. Also I think, just
maybe, that some of my taste is coming back! Things really do
seem to be getting easier . . . famous last words!

Just writing this morning and Dr Hasan just came around
with the old consultant whose name I do not know. It was really
moving. I really don't think I'll be able to explain why, it's kind
of like a. . . a. . . oh I don't know. . . a journey's reminiscence. . .

You know like at the end of some films, or series, it flashes
through the highs and lows of the entire story/episodes? Like
when, clip-by-clip, it goes through images of all that's passed in
a short time? Like the ending of 'To Kill a Mocking Bird' for
example. Well, it was kind of like that in a strange way.

He asked about my journal and I said how pleased I am that
I have kept it. He asked what are the main points in it and I said
about my old heart and the emotion of saying goodbye to it and

how it remained a paradox – extremely ill and bad, yet magnificent as well.

I told him about the gym yesterday – and how, for the first time, I could keep going; I caught us both really smiling. He said about telling Dr Reece. He told me to write in the letter I said I was going to write, 'Asif says congratulations on nurturing such a large heart.'

I just couldn't stop smiling and neither could he. I said it's going so well and I'm just so pleased. He said that I need to be here on Monday the 24th to meet and talk to some people – perhaps other colleagues ... I don't know.

A few days back Amanda said about the discussion – well, argument she said – to admit me to The Freeman to wait for the transplant. Amanda said they had others who were possibly needing admission and that some of the team wanted to do them first – I imagine it must always be a constant battle for the doctors to have to decide who they call and who they admit ... But Amanda said that the whole team thought I could sail through transplant, due to my unique condition (heart being extremely poorly and dangerous yet the rest of my body remaining largely asymptomatic).

She said the whole team thought I should do very well and it's rare for them to be presented with such a set of circumstances: a heart transplant on someone who does not have too severe heart failure symptoms. So they all had high hopes for me – perhaps higher than most patients, I think.

And this is kind of the feeling I got from Dr Hasan when he was just here. It's like they are as assured and buoyed by me and how I am, as I am indebted and grateful to them. It's almost like they kind of need me – or someone like me – as much as I, indefinitely, need them. They have given me a new heart and a new life – they chose me for it, and it's nice to know that in return I have achieved this recovery, so far, for them. Am pleased that, so far, I've given them the 'sail through' transplant that they and me, needed.

It wasn't an ending; am sure I'll see much more of Dr Hasan, but there really was something special about this visit.

I am in awe of Dr Hasan. He says very little indeed, but I truly believe he is one of the great men to have ever touched my life; I truly, truly do. Truly remarkable.

I don't want to write too soon, I really don't, but the fog is definitely lifting. I really am feeling more and more myself; today more than ever. My hands are shaking more now though which isn't very nice – especially to the reader! But my head, my poor-poor head is coming back! Almost totally back I would say ... brilliant.

Oh but my neck line is pulling really bad today. Have asked the nurse to put some more tape over it, but because I'm now on a ward, getting that done takes 30 minutes, if not more; also with the need to remind the nurse. Otherwise I'd be in the day room, or Chapel. But am just waiting here for a poxy piece of tape. Would rather just do it myself. Oh well, those sorts of irritations are testament to how well I'm feeling.

*   *   *

Midnight. Next day. My hand has completely stopped shaking all of a sudden. Completely. Hand-writing is still terrible because am writing in the dark. But no more trembles. None. Half way through my second blood-transfusion. Maybe that was it. How lovely ... Sleep now –

Day 13 – 15/05/2010

Well apologies for the rude interruption there above. Gushed out blood-transfusion without even giving the background. My hands have stopped shaking now though – let's see if you can tell the difference in the handwriting.

Well let's catch up with the rest of yesterday first. In the end

I asked another nurse for a roll of tape to secure my neck line [I.V taps] more – and then me and Mum high-tailed it outside.

Now let me just say something about going outside at the moment. Because they are building the 'Institute of Transplantation' at the hospital, the hospital is officially classed as a building site and certain air-particles, dissipated by construction work, can infect the lungs; there is a specific substance which is the villain, but I don't know what it's called.

So, because of the increased risk of infection, all Freeman hospital windows are taped shut. Every last one of them... well, except for my old cubicle on Ward 30 where, over time, I managed to push it back open!

Anyway, this all matters because when I go outside I am meant to wear a face mask. Well give-over! At the front of the hospital, in the little court-yard, the air could not be fresher. So I canned the mask – much to Pam and Mum's displeasure. I am allowed to be out in the fresh air without a mask, but the air at the Freeman is considered demolition grade ... and I'm sorry – it's just not!

But – and here's the thing – this very issue goes right to the heart of the journey my new life will take. And the issue is how much precaution should I take in light of my heart transplant and suppressed immune-system risks.

Should I panic every time I say hello to someone with a cold? Should I just run off? Should I obsess about washing my hands all of the time? Should I not go out in direct sunlight, even for 5 minutes without factor 50+ (Anti-rejection drugs mean I need a factor 50 when exposed to sunlight, due to increased risk of cancer)? Should I not eat Patè again? Should I not order dodgy take-away food again? (Food bacteria would naturally affect me more because of lowered immunity).

I mean I must just say that it 'is' really important, in the first three months, when my immune system is at its lowest to avoid germs; people who are ill, crowded places, supermarkets, swimming pools, work and so on, but after three months you can do anything.

However, within that freedom, being a transplant patient, you have to exercise certain cautions ... never allowed to wash with sponges/flannels, or soap bars, because they stay wet and harbour germs. I could go on and on ... however, the point I'm making is that all transplantees have to find their own way to respect and mind the risks, but also to live and enjoy life. And it is this line that needs drawing and it needs to be decided, straight away, exactly where it needs to be drawn.

It's nothing more than confidence on one side and respect on the other. You see I do not have much respect for the notion that the air outside the Freeman is bad, so, I decided, to draw the line there and trust myself – have confidence in myself, that I was okay.

I bet when Mum reads this she rolls her eyes thinking that confidence would soon become blaséness, or irresponsibility.

But, as I said, it's up to every transplantee to decide where the line that separates these things should be drawn. And building confidence up in my new heart, I think, is just so, so, so important. Let me say so far the things I have done to build my confidence...

Now, in the last two days only, I have locked the door when going into the toilet; before I was nervous that, if something happened, no one could get to me if the door was locked, so I just left it open.

Upon moving to Ward 25 they took me off of telemetry (heart rhythm monitor that broadcasts wirelessly to the nurses station's computer) and put me on a 3-lead stand alone monitor. If there's a problem it alarms, however, this is cumbersome, so when wandering around I disconnect myself from it. Yesterday it got to about 5 PM and I realised that I hadn't reconnected myself to the heart monitor. I then decided not to. Am sure if it was real important they would have reminded me, however, when I consciously decided not to plug myself back in, I started to doubt my heart beat ... was it dropping? Was it slowing? And I knew, in that moment,

I had to decide where to draw the line. I just relaxed and forgot about it.

See? I'm building confidence in my new heart already. But it's going to be an ongoing process – and one which I will not always get right.

Well, enough of that, let me tell you about another abating side-effect ... MY TASTE!!! Starting yesterday, through to this evening, that dreadful, metallic poison at the back of my throat ... has gone! And with that, back has come my appetite.

I am craving food again ... Pepperoni Pizza, McDonalds, eating out with Pam, Chinese, Indian, the lot. I wolfed down my dinner; Mulligatawny Soup and Sweet and Sour Pork with rice and an hour later I fancied more. I ate some Thorntons, grapes, Chedder's with smoked cheese – oh it was so nice to want food again.

My mouth is still quite dry – so not completely back to normal, but so, so much better. I have said this a few times today and sort of winced a little bit with that, 'tempting fate' feeling, but, even so, I'm still going to write it anyway: I really feel like I've turned a corner today. I feel more like my old-self than ever.

However, that was a little short lived as a little later one of the doctors came round and said I needed a blood-transfusion! I was taken aback because to me it sounded something really serious and that something must be quite wrong. Anyway, Pam went and asked Sister Ali and she explained it really, really well. She said that it is common for transplantees to need a blood-transfusion 1-2 weeks after surgery. The shock and trauma to the body means that to heal, you need to use your red blood cells – haemoglobin. But, because there is so much to heal, your bone marrow can't keep up with the amount needed, so they just give you a boost. Very, very common. Ali said that I should feel even better tomorrow, because a low red blood count makes you feel tired and lethargic. Well, I feel like that, but that's because I'm 13 days post-transplant I thought.

So that night I had 2 units infused and had my most awful, terrible, horrible night's sleep. I had the worst headache – over my eyes and over my forehead – that I've ever had. The lights didn't go off until midnight and my eyes were stinging. Then the lights kept going back on and my head just stung.

Tossed and turned, tossed and turned. At 4.30 AM I called Pam in tears; I was in so much pain and discomfort. She told me to get an eye mask from my bag – which I did. I soaked it in cold water and put it on... cold and dark... glorious!

I then fell straight asleep. Not sure if the headache was down to the light/sensitive-eyes, or the pain killer I dropped yesterday (Nefepan), or maybe something to do with the blood-transfusion? Who knows? It's morning now and the headache has gone – think it was all to do with my sensitive eyes.

Still, this morning, although my headache has gone; my body – upper body, shoulders, chest and back – is really tender and sore. Not sure if it's because I tossed and turned all night, or again because I've dropped that strong pain killer. It's not too bad though.

My shakes have almost completely gone as well – as you can tell by how much I've written this morning, which is so good. So, major gripes gone are:

Foggy head	–	Gone
Iron taste	–	Gone
Dry mouth	–	Still present
Foreign-body feeling	–	Gone
Hum in the ears	–	Gone
Central line pulling on neck	–	Hopefully gone tomorrow

Things really are on the mend. And I can really see that light, at the end of that tunnel.

Day 14 – 16/05/2010

Well, I was premature with a few things I wrote yesterday. One, my shaking didn't completely go; it was still slight, but got worse throughout the day. This morning it's not too bad – not gone, but quite bearable; just makes writing a little more effort. Also, for a large chunk of yesterday I felt quite rubbish. So, so tired and heavy and knackered. Was frustrated and irritable as well. Pam, as ever, bore the brunt of it with grace and patience and love. So, I just stayed in bed from about midday to about 6 PM. Felt tired enough not to be able to even get up – I could . . . I just felt well tired. Probably because of the awful night's sleep the night before.

Pam got me Domino's Pepperoni Pizza for lunch. It was such a struggle for her. She walked Alex home at 12-ish because he was really ratty when we were sitting outside in the courtyard. Then, because Mum wasn't around, Pam, with Alex constantly crying and grizzling, ordered the pizza, got Alex in and out of the car whilst it was raining, went to get it and then drove it over to me – and we sat in the car and ate it.

It was well nice – still not tasting completely the same, but a lot better. I was moaning at Pam on the phone, complaining about the time it was taking and where I was going to eat it and what's going to be done with Alex.

All that and the stress of Alex crying in her ear constantly and she still got me a pizza and brought it over and didn't complain, or moan once. She is just amazing. Mum was meeting a friend-of-a-friend in Newcastle for the morning – think she's finding it hard up here being cut off and isolated; that's why she wanted to meet up with this counselling friend-of-a-friend.

But Pam though has just been wonderful; everyday, every visit, every moment. She has been there for me completely, inexorably, resolutely, compassionately, lovingly, caringly, peacefully, silently, metaphysically . . . She has been there, by my side, keeping me strong, in every way anyone could ever be.

There is nothing more, since Neil came into my room, at 1.30 AM, two weeks ago today, that Pam could have done for me. There is not one aspect, one detail, part, one little bit of anything that she hasn't done to a perfect, 100% amount. For in these two weeks she has shown care and support which makes me cry just to think about it...

That woman is a wonder. As important and integral as my medicines and hospital doctors. Oh Pam, I just love you so, so much. So, so, so, so, so much... and Alex –x–

When I was slobbing about yesterday in a down mood I re-read what Mum and Pam wrote during Theatre and I.C.U. I'm so, so pleased they did that. Am so pleased. What Pam wrote was so lovely;

'*You are fine, you are safe, you are here,*
You are mine, you are Maxwell.'

Oh my eyes flood with tears instantly, no matter how many times I read that. I just can't hold back the tears. And when Mum wrote;

'*Watching Pam with you, Max, is such a delight. She immediately goes to you – not put off by any of the paraphernalia – and strokes and kisses your face and brow, whilst uttering such gentle words of praise and love and care.*'

Oh I can just picture it; Pam, pouring all her love and strength and spirit over and into me in I.C.U. Flooding my ears with her voice. Singularly wrapping my very core in her bare, honest love and crushingly pulling me back up, back to life – back with her.

I can picture her over me, connected to my new heart, more than the pacing wires. I can see her flood into me, more than the intravenous medicine and permeate my whole body; down to the place that only she knows exists, because it's only her that has ever been there. I can just picture this in my mind. And that is why – I just know this to be true – that is why, whilst still under full sedation, I opened my eyes. It's rare to do that. They usually start lowering the sedation before you respond, but even with no sedation decrease – I opened my eyes.

And I know why, because to begin with the sedation was just keeping me unconscious. But when, as Mum wrote, Pam came over to me and started kissing and talking to me, and infused into me, and flooded down to that spot which I just mentioned, well, then we were back together again; and the sedation could not keep us both under.

You see it's not that I could hear Pam and that gave me the strength to open my eyes – no. It's that Pam flooded inside me and immediately adopted my new heart and the pair of us, in essence, opened my eyes; beating the unreduced sedation.

And since then Pam has stayed in that deep place – where she was before and will be forever more…

*   *   *

Man, today my hands have started to shake more than ever – it's really not bothering me that much though. I know it will eventually go. Towards the end of yesterday I picked up a bit and played the piano with Mum for…

[*Mum transcribing what I am dictating*] – Mum inscribing for me…

[*Me back writing instead of dictating to Mum*] – And that's how long that lasted! Because I'm shaking so much more today, Mum said that she would write for me exactly what I said. However, I said, 'Mum writing for me…' and she wrote what's above, 'Mum inscribing for me.' Within two words she had ad-libbed, she had imprinted some of her, into what I wanted to say. Believe me I know it wasn't intentional – it was just a natural instinct, however, I said 'no Mum', you have to write <u>exactly</u> what I say.

I asked her to cross it out. She refused. Then I said carry on then and started saying about the error and Mum refused to transcribe it. She said why can't I just let it go. Don't think she realised that if within two words she had, unintentionally, deviated from what I explicitly said, she would have naturally carried on doing so the whole time, unless I made such a fuss about the very first mistake.

Precedents you see. Precedents are amongst the most important of things. It's precedents that turns a window-breaker into a hardened criminal, a wonderful town into a dive and vice-versa, a one kiss mistake into an adulterer and maybe, what's more important to me, a few misplaced doubts into complete paranoia and fear of life.

Anyway, enough of that. Let me just say that Mum more than made up for the minutes-taking-error, by suggesting writing with a pencil. She said it would be easier, so, as you can see, we bought some from the shop and I tell you, it is so, so good. So, so, so much easier to write with. I can still write fast and it be legible – am well pleased.

So back to what I was writing on the page opposite. I picked up in the evening and played the piano for quite a while – this bloke came into listen. He didn't want me to stop. He said that when I played it reminded him of home – he was Polish; a hospital worker, not patient.

Anyway then, a little later, I went on the bike on 27A. Didn't push myself too much though – just done 10 minutes on level 2, but dropped down to 1 after 3 or 4 minutes; there are no points for rushing my muscles – I must remember that ... I must.

Anyway that felt really good and then I got the nasty bright light in the ward, turned off – sure that's what my headache was all about. I put my eye mask on and took a sleeping tablet (ooh here comes dinner) and slept in lumber: All. Night. Long.

Heaven.

WEEK **8**

Day 15 – 17/05/2010

Second biopsy! Was much the same as the first; quick, but this time I walked down to the screening room – light headedness has completely gone! Anyway get the results tomorrow, however, the best thing about it – and I'm going to imitate screaming by how large I write this next bit; the larger the writing, the louder and more meaningful and significant it is . .

MY NECK CEN- TRAL LINE IS OUT!!

And it just feels so, so good. So free. So, so free. I can turn my head at will without thought, without fumbling around with the I.V taps – without a pull in the side of my neck ... Heaven. I seem to be writing that word more and more, recently.

A metasystem's analysis over the past three days' writing will tell you that I'm getting better by the truck load.

Today, played the piano, sat outside with Pam, then Mum – had a little workout in Ward 27A – played Connect-4 with Pam and lost – and then played Ludo and won; well, was going to win, but the nurses wanted their kitchen back, so we had to cut it short. However, the result was a forgone conclusion [*Pam's writing*: (Wishful thinking Max!)]

I have two more things to write about today, however, my hands are shaking wildly and they are also starting to cramp up, so I'll leave it until tomorrow night.

Oh I can't wait to tell you about one of them ... and the other; I can.

Goodnight –x-

Day 16 – 18/05/2010

Start with the good news.

Yesterday Sister Ali, whilst I was on the bike in 27A, come over to me and Pam and said, '*right Max, the plan for you is biopsy result tomorrow, Outpatients introduction appointment at 2 PM, my L.A line* (small tube into my left-atrium – which is bandaged up) *will come out...*' then she said '*... and we will be looking to discharge you after that.*'

I may be discharged TODAY!!! As long as all the paper work and tablets from the Pharmacy and a last little review of their transplant-training, can all get done in time – oh, and obviously the biopsy result has to be okay too – then I can go back to the house. TODAY!

Can you believe it? When she told us, I just got off the bike and gave Pam a quick cuddle; we were both beaming from ear-to-ear. Of course nothing is ever certain, but how cool is that!

The other thing is about another patient; Michael. When we were turfed out of 27A into the bay on Ward 25, two beds down from us was Michael. Not sure how old he was. I reckon around 40ish – could be younger, could be older.

Anyway I spoke to him a few times. He was waiting for a heart transplant too. He was here until he got one. The brief story he gave us of himself was that he'd been on the heart transplant list for nearly 4 years. However, at the start of his condition (don't know what the condition was) he wasn't too bad, but has been slowly deteriorating over the last few years.

He became so ill a year ago he had a V.A.D (Ventricular Assisted Device) – a mechanical heart fitted; lots of people are having them – you just have a wire coming out your side, plugged into a bum-bag type device, which you carry around everywhere.

However, four days after he had the V.A.D fitted, it gave him a stroke and he lost most of the use of his right-side: swallow reflex, arm movements, hand movement. Over the last year, from the stroke to now, he's learnt to write with the other hand and has painfully – through physio – gained a lot of his right-side function back. He was showing us that he can, only just recently, touch each fingertip on his right hand with his thumb.

His speech, he said, is a lot better, but he still finds it difficult. He doesn't really stutter, just talks quite slowly and pauses, thinking of the word, for awhile. He has been here for 5 weeks waiting so far. His family live a long way away, so he is by himself up here in general – although I'm sure they come to visit.

Mum asked him if he read books. He said the stroke has made him dyslexic, so he can't really read anymore. Apparently he used to be in the Air Force.

Around last year – when he was at home still working – he started to catch real severe infections, which made him too ill for transplant. After about the fourth large infection, they decided that the only way he could be transplanted, was if they kept him in hospital, with lots of antibiotics, to get him well enough for it.

But, the most overriding thing, other than his story, is the way he looked and spoke; very thin, gaunt, hunched – slightly hollowed eyes – real slow speech, but you can tell he's yearning to talk quicker. He spoke of his active days when he was in England's Boomerang team at the International Championships. He said he was going to cry if he kept talking about it, because it's been so long since he could do anything like that, that it just makes him so upset. He said how bored he gets here – wanders around to talk to the staff, but he says they're busy and can't talk for long.

The thing is, when I saw him, thin and frail, I had an over-whelming sense of pity. And I didn't like myself for it. I don't know why. To pity someone, although I couldn't help it, feels a little … a little … disrespectful? Perhaps. Am not sure really. Compassion is a wonderful thing, but just bare pity, it's not very nice. And I didn't feel nice about it.

Saying that though, the only way I can feel comfortable with the amount of pity I have for him, is that alongside that malignant pity, burns an electric hope of a return to FULL health. And this is the most overriding and enduring aspect of transplantation therapy; a chance – a hope – of no matter how ill you are, how dire the situation, how pitiful and painful the before has been and for however long – there is always – ALWAYS – this burning, searing hope of complete health again.

Hope really is, perhaps, one of the most important things we can have. And that's what I was saying to Mum. I suppose I pitied him so much, because I know I could, because I knew he had so, so much hope. But you could tell in his eyes and his manner and his body, that he has really suffered, that he really has gone through so much pain and struggle – you could really tell it in him; his mood was depressing, not really depressing, but he was never chirpy. It was more like he was really tired, in body and spirit it seemed. So sad.

Then, two days ago now, at about 7 in the morning, Ann (another transplant co-ordinator who I haven't really met) came round to Michael and said they have an offer on a heart which looks good for him.

The heart was good and he was taken down to Theatre at about 1.30/2 PM. But all the morning he was talking on his phone to lots of different people. I had the impression he was a loner, as he had no visitors, but that wasn't the case at all. He spoke to what sounded like close friends, close family and many more. He was so pleased.

With transplants, you are told about the offer of the organ and that it looks suitable – then there's a certain amount of hours that pass, where the recovery team perform lots of tests on the donor organ and loads and loads of blood work goes off and comes back, bit by bit.

Therefore, the more time that passes without it being cancelled, the better and more certain it is that the transplant will go ahead. So as the hours passed, he grew in excitement. I heard him say on the phone he's been waiting for this for 4 years and now he's fit and healthy, he's ready for it and can't wait. He said because they have kept him well in the hospital and infection free, he has no worries about the surgery. He must have said to about half-a-dozen people that he couldn't wait to get back into life and living again.

When he first saw me, when I came over from 27A and I said that I had my transplant 12 days ago, he was really impressed at how well I was doing, so fast too. He said a few times to the people he was talking to on the phone, *'There's a lad here who's had it done less than two weeks ago and already he looks ready to take on the world, so hopefully I'll recover like him.'*

As he was saying bye to everyone he was saying, *'love you,'* and *'don't worry'* and *'we'll be back doing this and that again before long.'* He said that he was so thrilled and excited. The shadowy gauntness and slightly pitiful look had gone and he was smiling quite a bit. I didn't say bye when the porters came – I wasn't there and when I left the ward he was in the shower, so I didn't get a chance to wish him good luck. But the heart in the end was good (he's had a few false alarms before which really got to him), so at last it was a good heart and the wait was over.

Michael didn't survive the surgery. The new heart wasn't taking well and was not working properly, so, after quite a few hours of surgery, they decided to withdraw.

I was so upset. I could have easily cried. All that pain, all that suffering, all that struggle, for so, so long for, in the end, when the heart finally comes, it all to go wrong.

I would never say all that suffering was for nothing – because nothing is for nothing – but it's just so sad. Life. Death. Me juxtaposed to Michael – there must be something to all of this… there just must be.

Apparently the nurse said he had a young family – God be with them … please. I can still vividly picture him and that pity I felt and his joy and elation when he knew he was having the transplant.

I suppose at least he died happy, content and hopeful – 'at least????' Huh, what am I saying…

Day 17 – 19/05/2010

Now I'm going to write about the time from the morning of the 18/05 to this morning the 19/05; 24 hours, which, among so many events and experiences, were probably the most amazing, wonderful, overwhelming, uplifting, happy, blissful, sincere, perfect, moving, life-changing, positive, awesome 24 hours of my life so far. So much so, that I am, for once, at a complete loss to know how to write about it ... to know where to start.

Just where do I begin to tell you about the joy, the other-worldly, impossible joy and happiness and wonderment, that I have experienced in the last 24 hours? Thinking about it makes my hands shake more than the Cyclosporin side-effects ... it really does.

I'll tell you what it feels like. It feels like every Guardian Angel, every God from every religion, every force of nature, every prayer from the four corners of the earth, every part of all the heavens and every effect of divinity and providence from across the whole universe have all, all, come together and in one omnipotent group consciousness, for some reason – a reason I'm sure I'll never, in this lifetime, be able to fathom – have decided to concentrate all that infinite power onto and into these 24 hours of Max Crompton's life.

I just can't believe the amount of goodness that I and my family have been blessed with, over the past 24 hours. This day could be used as a control day for the whole world to compare its individual happiness against – such is its essence and most virgin joy. I just can't believe it all rained down on me. I just really can't.

What have I done, what could I possibly have done, that could, in any way, deserve this? Well, you're probably getting irritated at me writing about the event's effects and not the events themselves ... so here goes...

Was pottering about the ward in the morning, awaiting the all important biopsy results and Pam called. She is pregnant. Normally saying this next bit would be a bit crude, however the nature of the situation up here in Newcastle, I think, precludes any taboo. You see we slept with each other just once – in our home-away-from-home, on the only afternoon we were alone; Mum, Alex and John had walked into Newcastle for the afternoon. (27/04/2010)

Even though Alex is really young, me and Pam know more

than most the importance and preciousness of time, and even with a successful heart transplant, life longevity, on balance, is not as great as 'normal' people, so we had, long before we came up to Newcastle, started to try for another baby. Heart transplantation is a risky business and if the worst would have happened, the second child we naturally wanted, would not have been able to have been.

Anyway, our trying for a baby was hampered, it seemed; Pam took a long time to recover from childbirth, then she was unwell with her thyroid, which took a while to stabilise. Then she was critically ill in intensive care with Toxic Shock – I still can't believe the way of the world. So it seemed it was fated that we would have to go through the transplant before trying for another.

But, this morning, on the phone to Pam, whilst I was pottering about the ward, I learnt that we were meant to conceive. All the time during the wait for theatre on that Monday morning, all the time Pam was playing with Alex whilst I was being operated on, all the time in I.C.U and 27A and Pam was pregnant! We were, technically, four – not three.

And then another thought struck me. That enduring image I pictured in my mind, as the anaesthetist was just about to take me away, of me and Pam and Alex, all cuddling in a tight embrace… well, thinking about it, there was a fourth person there; a fourth member of my family held in that enduring, everlasting embrace. How wonderful. What wonderful, wonderful news. She's around 5 weeks she reckons, so it's still really early days yet. But what timing … almost divine-like providence.

We really wanted another baby and at the hardest times of mine and Pam's life, when we were being tested the most, more than you can imagine … when things were just so hard – so, so hard – we were given this gift – along with the gift of a new heart and a new life … all within a few weeks. Pregnant, as well as a successful heart transplant with a supercharged heart [*Dr*

Hasan called the heart 'supercharged' as the heart was so strong and powerful] and a perfect operation and early recovery period and negative first biopsy result – awaiting second biopsy result.

Can you believe it? And whilst tumbling all this wonderment around in my mind in the early hours after Pam called, I realised that this baby was conceived with my old heart; my 'birth' heart, that has now been relieved of its struggle, that has now been laid to peace, after 27 years of gifting me a life that it had, according to the medical profession, no rights in giving me.

My thoughts become so poetic and romantic as I explore the meaning of it all … like my heart knew that it was soon to be laid to rest and as a parting gift, as a leaving memento, as an enduring legacy, it left a child. Now I know conception is the process of a different organ entirely, but it's all powered by the heart; it's all driven, firstly and ultimately by its constant beat. So, you can see how, romantically, I can place the first cause of conception at my birth heart's door; exclusively and totally. If I didn't think more highly, or magnificently of my heart before, it's hard not to be utterly in awe and bewildered at it now.

I am now to move onto a new life, with a new heart; and what a perfect thought to bear at the crossroads of this junction – that my birth heart, in its last main act, gave us a second child, before it was removed, to finally be at peace… at rest … its job – finally done.

God bless and Goodbye -x-

That is only up to the afternoon. There's still so, so much more in this 24 hours.

At 2 PM we went for our introductory out-patients appointment. There, Mary told me that my second biopsy result came back showing zero rejection. What unbelievably wonderful news. She then went through out-patient procedures and said my first appointment is in two days time; blood test, E.C.G and chest X-ray is what it comprises of. An hour or two, tops.

Then went back to the ward and, after having my L.A line out (left atrium wire) and a quick chest X-ray to check that removing it from inside the heart caused no damage – which it didn't – I was officially DISCHARGED! Inpatient stay 30/03/2010 – 18/05/2010; 48 nights, 49 days. So, so much passed, in, when you think about it, such a small amount of time.

Me and Pam packed up my bags and I walked out of the Cardiothoracic block's main entrance a free man, not a Freeman inpatient! Mum and Alex, by timing's coincidence – or fate, I'm sure, considering all of this – walked up to the hospital just as we were discharged. And we... crap... missed out something incredibly important in this 24 hour, chronological diary. I'll interject it now and then return to outside the Cardiothoracic block.

Whilst I was milling around the ward, waiting for my X-ray results to let me go home, I ran into Kirsty on 27A. She said that she had some brief donor details. We went into 27A's kitchen and she told me that his name was Andrew and that he was rushed to hospital with a bleed in the brain; a brain haemorrhage.

He was 35 years old, in perfect, full-body health. No symptoms, no condition, no medical problems and then, all of a sudden, a weak blood vessel burst in the brain and he was rendered brain-dead. No pain, no warning, no time experiencing anything – just perfectly healthy one moment and dead the next; body being kept perfused by a ventilator.

Kirsty explained how much the donor process means to the bereaved family. She said that years ago things like this just happened and it's awful. Now they happen still and it's still just as awful, except now, out of such misery, 1, 2, 3, 4, 5, or even more people could be saved from perpetual suffering. And Kirsty said that the bulk of donors are where there has been brain bleeds, or brain related illness. It's only really the Neurological departments where transplant liaisons work – which we know from Dad, all too well.

Anyway, I said to Kirsty that in due time, not now, but not in too long-a-time, I will write a letter to the donor family – once it's written, I will put a copy in this journal.

Later on, me and Pam decided that the baby's middle name will be Andrew if it's a boy and Andie if it's a girl, as a mark of remembrance and respect to Andrew and Andrew's gift, that I have received. Anyway, that happened before discharge – now I'll return to outside the Cardiothoracic block; me, Pam, Mum and Alex, ready to walk back home ... to stay!

It was about 5 PM. The sky was lidless; nothing but that blue that I wrote about in the first journal. The sun was soft and warm and permeating. It was like the weather had been divinely ordered to make the walk home as conducive to the feeling of peace and true freedom, that I was already feeling in moving from an 'In', to an 'Out', patient. Finally, I could spend the night ahead with my family, in my home.

For a lot of the ten-minute walk I strode a few paces ahead of the others, in a tranquil silence; a deep sense of stillness and gentle calm. I was awashed with a feeling of everything coming to a rest ... A macrocosm of unrest and change and movement, finally coming, not to an end, not by a long way, but for the time being at least, coming to a plain, simple, neutrality.

I felt so calm. It was utter bliss. Like ice-cold water, poured generously over your forehead when it's throbbing from staring into direct sunlight for too long. Heaven; that word again.

Being at home that evening , we ordered Chinese take-away. Me and Pam laid on the lovely comfy sofa and watched The Simpsons. I ate so much Chinese ... it was so, so nice. Have such an insatiable appetite of late. Not sure if it's because I'm returning to my old self and am making up for any lack of appetite since transplant, or if it's the steroids. Either way I couldn't have cared less – I just ate and ate and ate. And a few hours later, in bed, I was fantasising about having another plateful!

Sleeping with Pam again that night, was, just simply, in a two-worded phrase... coming home. And I really feel that I need say no more than that. Those two words really do say it all.

Then there was the morning. Alex, although slept like he was in hibernation throughout the night, woke up early at 5.30 AM. Secretly I was over-the-moon that he woke up then – I had long been awake, awaiting his little stirring voice. I would have loved to have gone into him when he woke to pick him up, but I cannot hold Alex at all really, at the moment. The small matter of a sternotomy gets in the way, but that puts me off surprisingly little – just seeing and being with him again is enough; I'll hold him again, all in good time. I suppose it frustrates me so little because it is literally too painful to hold him, it's not that I'm just not allowed to.

Anyway, Pam brought him in with us and we spent the first few morning hours, all snuggled in bed together. It was an identical, identical feeling to what I said in a reflection I wrote, on the 20/09/09, entitled 'Intensive Care Anniversary.' To save my shaking, cramping hand, Pam will transcribe the exert, for good measure...

Intensive Care Anniversary exert

This morning I laid lazily in bed ... with Pam and with our three-week-old, to-the-day, baby boy, Alex James... beautiful baby Alex, at the precise time, was laying snugly along my thighs, with our cover laying gently over him.

I had kinked my knees so he was laying at an angle facing me and Pam with the window behind pouring soft, autumnal morning light, warmly over his adorable face. He was as contented as could be – his inescapably large, navy-blue eyes, were darting back and fourth, up and down and with every new stare his little lips and ever podgier cheeks, moved through expression after expression, with a carefree abandon and randomness only possible with newborns.

Us three laid there for some time. I put our music on. And we just laid there, me and Pam, both staring at Alex with an intensity that he was, no doubt, looking out with also. The morning sun stayed constant and our brand new family were enjoying the empty minutes that were falling by without comment or purpose...

Thanks Pam, nice writing, although a little slanted ☺. In essence this morning was just like that. Obviously there are many literal differences; Alex being 8 ½ months old now and much more interactive are the main ones – but that feeling of empty minutes, falling by, is the main thing. The morning, was, yep – I'm going to use that word again; heaven. And that is the 24 hours.

Now I deliberately saved this next sentence until last – not because of its importance, far from it... actually... you know what... I'm not going to write it. No. Decided. It will not be penned. Only I will know it.

The reason I'm not going to write it is that this new life I'm starting is a dawn of many new things, but, perhaps, most paramount, it's the dawn of a greater certainty in my life. And in line with that, the sentence will not come to light.

That's the 24 hours done. Un-be-liev-able. Just simply unbelievable. I'll let my poor hand rest now. Bye.

Ooo, I have something wonderful to tell you about today – but I'll leave that until tomorrow

Day 18 – 20/05/2010

Now. Today I'm only going to write about only one thing from yesterday. And unlike yesterday's writing, I'll start with the event and then try, as best I can, to show, what it meant to me. I know I'll fail on that part, because, as Tom so wonderfully wrote in a letter to me once, words are for everyone and because only I can truly know what it feels like, whatever words I use to describe it, will, ultimately fail, because if they didn't, the whole world would know what everything is like for everyone – which we all know cannot be. So, by taking what it means into the realm of words, will ultimately be self-defeating, because it's the surest way to guarantee that the true meaning cannot come across.

However, my writing is my best tool and although far from perfect, describing the feeling will hopefully give you a vacant abstract echo, a barely audible whisper, of what it was like for me...

Opposite the hospital is Paddy Freeman's Park and as I said in Journal 1, there is a deep ravine down to a river and a little waterfall. To roughly gauge the depth of the dene, there are large, tall trees that stretch from the base, to around two-thirds up the ravine side. The descent down is a combination of steep slopes, shallows inclines and random runs of rough steps of varied height.

Looking at the descent with my birth heart, I doubted and feared, that if I went to the bottom, I not so much wouldn't make it back to the top – I'm sure, deep down, I would have – however, I feared about the state I would be in and the struggle it would put on me and my birth heart. I would only have been able to do it with a series of stops along the way; the stops becoming more frequent and for longer periods, the further I got up to the top. And indeed getting to the top would have really, really strained me.

Usually I would have still done it – investing monumental effort, excruciating fatigue, a burning throat, suffering a two-tonne body and that perpetual feeling of weakness and battle and pain to have gotten to the top. However, being an inpatient on the heart transplant waiting list, I was much more reserved and decided to save the ascent for my new life – if it came...

Well, as you already know, my new life has come and I

decided to put it to the test and go all the way down, to the bottom of the waterfall.

Now, before I go into it, I just want to give a little further perspective. I have already written about a Eureka moment in the gym, where I could do more, much more than I could ever have done before. However, what I'm about to tell you far, far surpasses that gym feeling, and I have realised – and it makes me shake when I realise this – that as I recover and grow stronger, this feeling that I will try to describe, these Eureka moments – so to speak – will keep growing in power... will keep on increasing in wonderment... will just keep on multiplying and multiplying and taking me higher and higher, until I am soaring away from my old self; soaring through the clouds in the sky, ascending up and up through the different atmospheres – out of this world and beyond. Until I reach a point, maybe not too far from now, where that sodden marshland of physical struggle, is a universe away.

Although what I am about to tell is monumental and life changing to me – it is merely the first few seconds after take-off, of the journey from those sodden marshland, to the furthest stretches of that new universe of possibility. So, back to the foot of the waterfall...

I stood on the small hump-backed bridge, over the flowing water, and, at normal walking pace – not brisk, but not slow – started walking. Right at the start there are around 7 high steps. I climbed them and was then on a shallow incline; not very steep at all. And, after a few paces on this shallow slope, I realised that my legs had, within 2 seconds, forgotten that they had gone up those steep steps and my body felt identical to when I had been standing on the hump-backed bridge. Needless to say that with my old life, I would have already been feeling the effects of those several steep steps – effects not just of calf and thigh strain, but of an increasing weight through the core of my body, shoulders, neck and head.

Anyway, the low gradient soon gave way to a steep incline. I continued to walk up it – the only feeling of anything happening was in my calves; I was conscious of their presence, nothing more. Then another run of about 10 steps, but these were very thin; no trouble at all.

Then, turning through 180 degrees in the zigzag path of the ravine side, I come to the guts of the ascent – one, continued, high gradient, steep hill, right to the summit. I walked. I just simply carried on walking – the same pace – much the same feeling; the feeling of nothingness everywhere, except by now, aching calves, slightly straining thighs and much heavier breathing.

My pace remained constant. Step by step, up and up and up and then without fuss, without a triumphant drum-roll relief, without a crushing feeling of reassurance that the ordeal was at an end, without a collapse onto the grass with arms folded over my head and body totally devoid of all physical and structural integrity. Without the joy of knowing that I had actually made it all the way up – without that background, almost sub-conscious feeling of real dysfunction... disability... weakness. Without that weight – that obtrusive, pervading weight that pulls on every bone, on every muscle in my body: like my blood had been replaced with wet cement – like two bowling balls had been suspended on two long wires attached to the corner-joints of my jaw – just behind my ear-lobes. Without that feeling of immediate physical imprisonment, in the early recovering minutes, when I'm collapsed on the floor. It's almost like, at the top, I'd have been like a tortoise, upside-down on its shell – stuck, but stuck by fatigue and impossible weight – weight which makes you think that Newton's laws of gravity were wrong – were surely too light.

However, as I was saying, I went up and up and up and reached the top... and... just stood there; out of breath, calves and thighs hot and slightly sore – and every other part of my body a feeling of... nothingness... normality. Like every other part of my body, except my calves and thighs, had been taken to the top by helicopter – like someone else took my torso and

arms and shoulders and neck and head up to the top for me ...
Surely it was not me that took them? Surely not...?

But it was. And I couldn't even feel that I had. It just felt like
the hill was a mirage... an optical illusion. It was really just a
gentle slope of a few hundred meters ... it must have been ...
surely? But again, it wasn't. It was me that ascended the ravine
– and the ravine was steep, was deep, was all the way down to
that waterfall.

And then something quite powerful happened. I was already
overcome with the physical feelings of what had just happened,
but then, like a gale, like an Atlantic rip-current, I filled with a
type of anger; a type of rage foreign to me. And instantly I knew
what I wanted to do...

I marched – back down – back down the ravine, back to that
same spot, on that same hump-backed bridge, at the waterfall's
feet, fiercely determined, to march back up a second time.

As I strode down in quick-step, I felt that very, very powerful
emotion build and build – exponentially – with every step back
down; every step which become quicker and quicker as the
feeling multiplied into – all I can call it, is a WRAITH.

It felt like, from the very first thing that I realised I couldn't
do – all those years ago – I started to scream at the thought, or
knowledge, at not being able to do it – probably run-outs, or
nursery playground chase – something like that. And since that
first memory of Ebsteins' limitations, that first scream has
continued – in the background – which, without thinking about
it, I didn't – day-to-day – know it was there. And that scream
that started then, has been added to, every time I've had to
stop early, every time I've had to retire from participating, every
time I've had to sit out, every time I have just simply not been
able to do something normal people could – every time I've felt
that suffocating heaviness, every time I've had to doubt myself,
every time I've approached an exertion with fear at not being
able – Every Single Fucking Thing that I have ever struggled
with, or physically been beaten by – all, individually, every

single instance, has added to that scream that started from that very first game of playground chase.

Over say 23/24 years the scream, which was always in the background, finally – on that march back down to the base – finally, finally showed itself to me . . . And I was awestruck. I saw this single resonating record of all of the pain and all of the struggle, manifested in this feeling I was now possessed with; this scream I could hear, tearing through the void. And I wanted to at last. . . Unleash It! Unleash all its fury, pain and terror onto this ravine – onto this second ascent.

I got to the bottom, took a deep breath, started my stopwatch on my mobile phone and this time marched – quicker than walking pace – heading back toward the summit again. But this time, with every step, the scream thundered through the earth, shook the trees, cascaded up the ravine like a monster. I felt like I wanted to murder the incline; kill it – with the scorch of this sickening scream. I tore up the hill like a thunderstorm, like a lion, like a helpless rage. All those years. . . all those things. . . all those times I couldn't – I manifested them all into knives and daggers to bludgeon and slice and stab the ravine into a bloody mess. I was possessed to defeat it – defeat it in so many ways and for so many reasons that I just cannot say.

The anger, the ferocity, the power of that pulsating scream raced me to the top again in 3 minutes 4 seconds. It was perhaps the most intense 3 minutes 4 seconds that I have ever lived.

At the top I was massively out of breath and both of my legs were burning like fire. But, I stood for a few minutes and after a short while – not too long – I walked off, again my body forgetting that anything had ever happened.

Unbelievable. I can't wait for tomorrow. And to think that this is just the first few minutes of that journey from those sodden marshlands, to the upper-reaches of that new universe of possibility . . . The whole thing makes me shiver to my core. The possibilities seem ceaseless.

What dreams really do come . . .

Day 19 – 21/05/2010

Yesterday I had my first Outpatient appointment of many. I got there at just before 8 AM . Had blood-pressure, blood test and weight done – which were fine – and then me and mum, who was with me, went to have a chest X-ray and E.C.G.

My E.C.G looks so standard now, so normal – because it is. It looks so different. I've now got a perfectly average heartbeat-trace that you can see below:

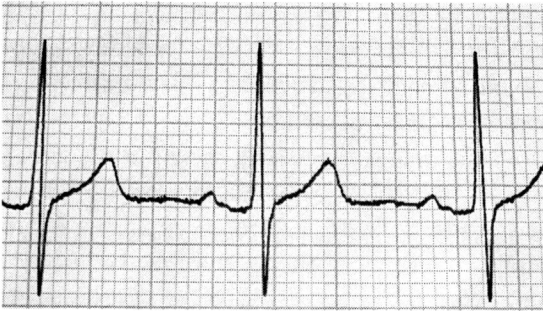

... two strong heart beats, right next to each other. My Ebsteins E.C.G was like this;

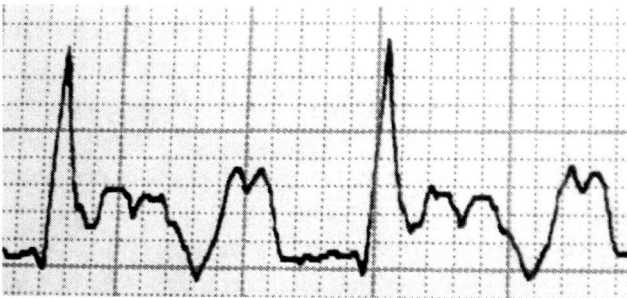

... two weaker heart beats, further apart and less amplitude. It's just so surreal seeing my E.C.G now.

Then we had a Full-Monty breakfast each whilst we waited until 10 AM for the Outpatient doctors. Saw Dr Bart, a small

Indian man who is really nice. He said that everything looks good and to call back at 3 PM for blood results and next outpatient's appointment and biopsy date.

Had to pick up my prescription and doctor's discharge letter from Ward 25. And, as I was walking along the corridor, I ran into Dr Choudhury and Amanda. You can tell in their faces how pleased they are to see me looking so, so well. Amanda said that on Tuesday Dr Hasan was quite disappointed as he came to see me to say congratulations about Pam, but we were away from the ward. How lovely is that. The UK's most accomplished Congenital Heart Surgeon – a man who attempts and completes operations that no one else in the country will do – took time to come all the way over to me to say congratulations. I'll definitely see him again before leaving, so that will be nice.

Dr Choudhury was really asking me what it's like, inside my mind – inside my soul were his exact words – knowing that I had someone else's heart. I tried to explain a bit, but said I would send him a copy of these Journals. He said if I publish them I could donate the proceeds to the transplant charity. Not a bad idea, but doubt I'll ever send this to any literary agents – but never say never.

The rest of the day me and Pam took Alex over the park for a few hours – it's the start of a three-day heat wave apparently – and then us three walked to Sainsbury's and back. I pushed Alex up the long, long slope back home without even noticing. In fact now, within reason, I am judging the steepness of any incline by my faculty of balance, rather than my feeling of fatigue . . . it's just such a wonder.

Then we popped to Asda to get a gazebo and sun-lounger for the garden, considering the Mediterranean weather we are having; don't want Alex to burn in the garden, or me not to be comfortable, lying like a commoner on the bare grass – I require something much more posteriorly gratifying!!! Check me out going to Sainsbury's and Asda in one day. Not sure if I'm reintegrating too much. They say with my immuno-suppression

I should slowly, bit-by-bit, reintegrate: for the first 6 weeks you should be really careful and then moderately careful up to 3 months; you can then go anywhere and do anything without reserve, but never – being a transplant patient – without caution.

Anyway both supermarkets weren't packed and you have to go through that 'risk' period when you just simply do not know if you've done wrong, or not – but, if nothing happens, then the confidence starts to build. And I'm fine so far; temperature this morning 36.4… excellent.

Had lovely undyed smoked haddock dinner and then went to bed with my gorgeous – with child – wife, for the third night on the trot … That feeling of 'coming home' has not worn off yet; we were parted for such a long time. So many nights I missed her touch… her scent… our 'spoonering'. It was so hard, but that makes these nights all the sweeter.

* * *

This morning [21/05/10] was like we had woken up in Puerto Banus, or Taormina … the weather … the morning … utter perfection. Blue skies, stingingly bright sunshine and a clarity of vision as intense and exact as a laser diamond cutter – as clear as a glass of ice cold mineral water – as pure as a fresh-water rainforest brook.

Alex was up really early – awoke at 5 AM, but we got him up at 6 AM – so, come 9 AM he was quite ratty. So me and him, father and son, just the two of us – alone for the first time in probably a couple of months – went for an early morning walk around Paddy Freeman's Park. It was glorious. We circumnavigated an entire circuit of the park. It took almost 45 minutes and I enjoyed every second. I would like to say Alex did too, except a few times I tried to do some serious off-roading with the buggy over tree-root lined mud tracks and thickly overgrown, boggy land – and the lumps and bumps made Alex start crying! So I high-tailed it back to the tranquillity of the path, pretty sharpish. He then went to sleep.

But the light. Crystal. Razor sharp. I even sat down on the bench just to look around at the vista of endless trees, running around the panorama. I just kept thinking about Louis De Bernieres' description of the light in Kefelonia in, 'Captain Corelli's Mandolin'. I'm sure this morning is what he was writing about.

Anyhow got back, put gazebo up and chilled in the garden, in the shade, in the heat. Then, at lunchtime me, Mum and Alex packed a picnic and went to the dene, next to the waterfall, for lunch; Pam had a massage booked so couldn't come. Turns out she could have though, because she wasn't allowed to be massaged until she is past 12 weeks pregnant – shame, as she was really looking forward to it.

Anyway me and Mum had a lovely picnic: home-cooked ham-joint sandwiches with avocado and sweet onion relish, spicy warm chicken strips, warm boiled eggs, yoghurts, crisps, apple, blueberries, raspberries, pretzels, Kitkats, plum tomatoes and Vimto – a feast.

Then me and me alone, pushed Alex, in his buggy, with heavy nappy bag and picnic remnants, all the way to the top of the ravine – all by myself. Was turbo knackered at the top, legs and breathing burning, but I had done it. I was so proud. I said to myself, me, I, Alex's Dad, have just taken him, personally, up the hill. I have done something for him that I would have never-in-a-million-years, have been able to have done before. The very first thing that I have done for Alex which I couldn't do before. Of course he was oblivious to it – he was sparko – but I suppose children never really know what their parents really do for them – and that's what makes it so worth while.

Anyway it was a wonderful feeling to be able to 'do' for Alex, in a way in which I couldn't have done before.

Then, this evening, me and Pam went to Pizza Express. It was gorgeous. I ate like a horse, but I am doing more physical activity now than I have ever done before, so it's not surprising I'm so hungry. Mmmmnnnn Romana-based, Sloppy Giuseppe pizza ... to die for.

And that pretty much brings me to the here-and-now ... these very strokes of pencil, still controlled by a shaking, cramping hand. Ooo guess what? Emma is coming up tomorrow for a night; yay! Can't wait to see her – and I can't wait for her to see me!

Night -x-

Day 20 – 22/05/2010

Awoke to another Andalusian-like morning. It's glorious out there. Mum, Pam and Alex are going to pop to Asda and I'm going to have a little time by myself here – will probably walk over to the hospital to play the piano. We're going to have a BBQ later in the garden when Emma gets here, but firstly I've been meaning to glue/add some stuff into this Journal.

I have had a few lovely cards from Auntie Carol and Tom's Lou and so on, but I will not glue cards into this Journal – I'll just put them in a keep-sake box with these Journals and I.C.D and any other transplant memorabilia. However, there are two exceptions:

Firstly what Pam's mum – Pat – sent me. She sent me printed emails she had received from her friends and family which were about me. In short, she has sent me people's thoughts and prayers and wishes, that they have had for me, Pam and Alex. It was so overwhelming receiving them. Everyone I talk to says that everyone is always asking about me and thinking about me and that certain people – church services – pray for me weekly.

All of this is wonderful; human kindness and caring at its most pure and natural – the soul showing its true face ... However, actually receiving the thoughts and prayers – what

Pat has sent – made me cry. Such a wonderful thing to do. I really am deeply, deeply touched. So here they all are [*family relation annotations are from Pat's perspective*]:

What a relief! – and, my prayer has been answered. I will continue to pray for a perfect recovery for Max. ~June x ~ **(Cousin)**

Hello Pat. Everything crossed at this end. Thinking of you all. I am sure everything will be ok in the end. Thank goodness they found him a heart at long last. Luv from Chris xxx **(Cousin)**

Dear Pat. Thinking of you and your special family. May all go well for Max and his amazing operation. How wonderful the family can stay near the hospital and Max's Mum is there to help Pam with Alex. Love, Viv **(School friend)**

Hope all is well Pat. Our thoughts are with Pam and family. XX Ann & Robin **(Work friends)**

Hello Pat. Great – everything seems to have gone well – thinking of you all. X Jackie **(Work friend)**

Dear Pat. What a relief for you all and fantastic news. Brilliant! Love Kerry **(School friend)**

Good news! I've said a prayer for Max – and Pam, baby Alex, the Surgeons, staff, and the other family of the heart donor – for a successful result. It must be all so stressful for you all, but Surgeons nowadays are doing such wonderful things. I shall be thinking of Max often for the next couple of months. Thank you for letting me know. ~June~ **(Cousin)**

Hi Pat. I have just read your email and would like to wish your son-in-law a speedy recovery. It must be such a worry for your daughter who herself has been ill recently. I hope she has fully recovered. My best wishes to them both. Speak soon. Elsi **(Cousin)**

*Good morning to you Pat. Many Thanks for the email. What lovely news! We are praying here that everything goes okay. It's a hell of a long time for an op, but I have a friend who will very soon be undergoing the same thing, when a suitable heart is found for her. Unfortunately, this is going to be a very anxious time for all the loved ones, but at least he will be given a further chance. Let's hope that everything goes according to plan and that it wont be too long before they are all back home as a family, and once again, altogether again. Our thoughts are with you all. All our love, from Lesley and Frank xxxx **(Ian's friends)***

*Dear Auntie Pat. Thanks for the update. Our thoughts are with Max, Pam, baby Alex and Uncle John. I hope everything goes well. I hope you are all ok under the circumstances. Love Sarah **(Pam's Cousin)***

*So pleased for you all **(Staff at Basildon Council)***

*Dear Patricia. After all this time...............we pray that everything proceeds satisfactory for them. Wonderful that they have rented a house so close to the hospital. It will no doubt give them a lot of confidence at the very beginning when it really does count. Let us know how things go and keep your chin up – they've come a very long way! Love Kerry and Pat. **(School mate)***

*Really pleased to hear the news about Max. It's a long haul now for him and Pam, but they have got everything on their side – I will say a little prayer for them. Thanks so much for letting us know. Love Val and Brian **(In-law relatives)***

*Hi, Hope all goes well. Will be thinking of you all, Luv Bren **(School friend)***

*Hi Pat, Fingers crossed, tell them all we'll be thinking of them. Karen xxx **(Cousin)***

*Pat, Many thanks for updates on Max's operation and later progress. Hope everything continues to go well. Best Wishes, Bill and Jenny **(Cousin)***

How wonderful. The other exception is a card/letter I got from Emma. Because it's more of a letter than a card – although part of it is a card – I think it merits an inclusion. Not sure how I'm gonna glue it in though!!? Oh well here goes – could do with a stapler!

Emma's Card & Letter

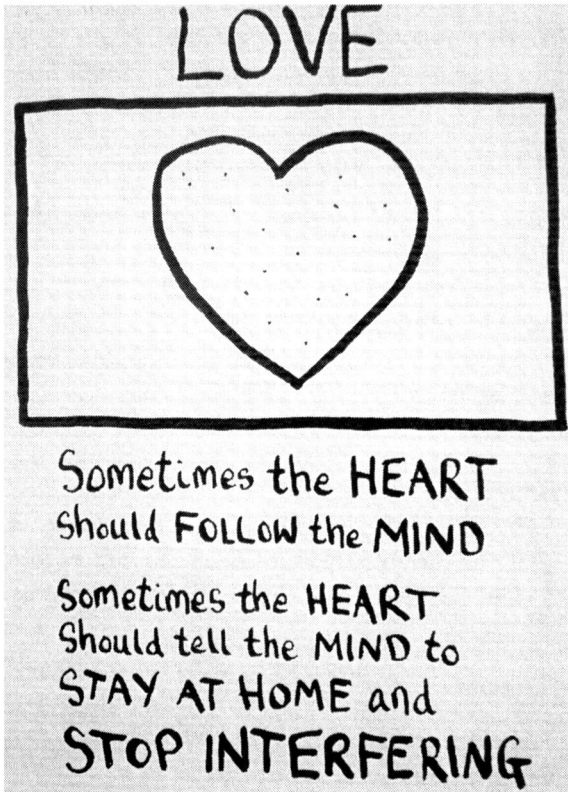

LOVE

Sometimes the HEART
Should FOLLOW the MIND

Sometimes the HEART
Should tell the MIND to
STAY AT HOME and
STOP INTERFERING

Dearest Max,

I have had this card for ages, and I have never really, as yet, managed to find a use for it (sorry you must think you're getting my 'cast-offs'!). Well now, I think it holds great meaning. Your heart, your 'old' heart that is (although there was nothing 'old' about it), in many ways, ruled your life, so one could say, it 'over-ruled' your mind too. By 'Mind', I mean to refer to your physical being. Therefore, despite all the physical evidence that your heart was failing, it endured, throughout it all. Your heart saw you through birth, your later harrowing operations, it guided you towards love, Pam of course, it again endured through your cardiac arrest & countless other procedures, ablations & ICD fitting, and then it found & held new love for the birth of your child, Alex. And so, as this card aptly says, the mind shouldn't interfere! The HEART, especially in your case, knows best, always has, and will continue to, too.

Anyway, wow, am still unable to digest all that has happened in the last 15 days. I am sitting in the morning sun, on one of my lovely chairs you bought us, with my cup of tea, and am trying to get my head around it.

Have thought a lot about Michael, such a sad thing. But as you said nothing (no suffering etc..) is ever for nothing, no reason. And I think in terms of me, what was the reason for me hearing it? Well, I think it was to make me realise the enormity of the transplant you have had. When something seems to go so 'smoothly' (of course you have had an incredibly hard journey but in terms of the operation, it went well) – it's easy to allow one's self to be comforted by the fact that transplants really are 'run-of-the-mill' at Newcastle, and rarely are any problems encountered. But of course, that's far too glossy-a-picture.

The other reason for me learning about Michael is, I think, to understand hope. The hope he felt, before surgery, was a good thing. He must have felt happiness again, happiness at all the possibilities that might have laid before him, hope that

*his 'old life' would become a reality once more. So, I truly
believe that HOPE, regardless of the outcome that follows, is
nothing but an extremely positive force. Jeez, it's doubtless the
human soul could survive without it. I heard a line recently
on a fairytale D.V.D I was watching with baby-Ben which
perhaps sums it up. The 'damsel in distress' is locked in a
tower by her wicked step-mother and remains there for years.
The narrator says "...although she was locked up, it's not true
to say she was a 'prisoner' for she had HOPE, and when you
have HOPE, you're never really anybody's prisoner".*

*And I think of you Max and all the events/things that you
could have allowed to hold you prisoner over the years. But
yet you have always had hope, as we all have for you, and so
your physical limitations have not enslaved you perhaps as
much as they would have if you had allowed yourself to be
ruled by despair.*

*Of course you have 'visited' despair, on a number of
occasions, but you have not remained there long. Jeez, and
now you are having another baby. Throughout all the
trauma of the last few weeks (48 days to be exact, if your
maths are to be trusted), your darling wife has been growing
another precious life. Your's and Pam's union is indeed a
marvel to behold. Such depth to your love of, and devotion to
each other. What an amazing thing for a baby to be born
into. Wow, still can't believe it all!*

*And of course, your donor! This guy, Andrew, the word 'thank-
you' barely scratches the surface of the indebtedness you, and
us, must feel towards him and his giving family. Bless them.*

*Well, I've rambled on long enough. Hope my writing has
been fairly legible!*
Love you Max-pax. Love you so very dearly.
See you soon hopefully,
Love Emma xxx

End of Emma's Letter

Also it evens it up a bit because I already have a letter from Tom and Lou wrote in Journal 1 and Mum and Pam have also contributed so now the card/letter from Emma, makes a full set! And whilst I'm in the mood for putting things in from others, below are texts Mum and Pam received whilst I was in theatre and the immediate hours after. However, before the theatre texts, Mum wants to include a text she sent to me a while ago:

Mum's text on 04/11/09 [*sent to me when we were at my second transplant assessment*]

There's nothing you can say that will make it ok,
There's nothing you can say that will make it go away,
There's nothing I can do that will make it better for you,
There's nothing I can see that will make it better for me.
But, if we put all that we have into a pot,
We will be reminded of all that we've got.
The strength and the courage to face the UNKNOWN-
Together with loved ones and on our OWN.
For although we can know nothing of what is to be,
We know it with SAFE UNCERTAINTY.
Like all episodes there's been,
We'll manage this one head on 'as a team'
(And there's no losers on our side)

End of Mum's Text

Below are a few texts I received during my op. At 1:36 PM 03/05 Pam sent this message: '*Max's op has gone well :o) The heart is working n they just stitching him back together, then they'll wheel him round to intensive care xxx*'

Trianda Replied: *Oh thank goodness. I'm so pleased, you must be so relieved! Thanks for letting me know Pam, Thinking of you all. Let me know when he is back if you can x*

Karen Replied: *Fantastic news babe. Hope the recovery's a speedy one. Big hugs n kisses.*

Al Replied: Fan-bloody-dabby-doesy, give my fav brother in law the biggest hug from me. Had a few words with the top man upstairs with a few amens, and he will be tip top. All our love, keep me updated x

Pedgy Replied: He is one in a million and we're all so lucky to have him in our family xx

Becky Replied: Hey Pam, great to hear the op went well … Thinking of you all up there. Hope to be back to Newcastle soon to see you all. Love from Becky. Gemma sends her love too xxx

Pam's Mum Replied: When he wakes give him a cuddle and big sloppy kiss from all of us xxx

Joyceline Replied: Praise be to God. This is FANTASTIC News!! Wishing him a quick recovery xxx

Wattsy Replied: This is excellent news. I'm so pleased for Max, you and Alex. Let him know we are all thinking of him and when the time is right for him, I'll come & pay him a visit. Keep me updated with his progress.

Pam then sent this next message at 9:48 PM the same day: *'Max is doing fantastic! He is off the ventilator breathing for himself and talking. Tomorrow hopefully they'll be moving him to H.D.U. He has done amazingly well, so proud of him.'*

And she then sent a third message at 11:35 AM on the 04/05: *'Max is fully awake this morning and laughing and joking. They are really pleased with his progress and plan to get him out of bed into a chair later today.'*

Eddy Replied: That's excellent news am so pleased for you guys. Tell him he can cut his own damn grass soon the lazy git ha-ha.

Wattsy Replied: Wow, that is excellent. I can't believe he's already awake and joking about. So pleased! I'll let the guys here all know as they've been asking after him.

Trianda Replied: *can't believe how well he is doing so soon! Supermax ;O) So pleased.*

Texts received on Mum's phone:

Emma: *Just called to see how max is doing. Feel such an over powering urge to c him. Know I can't and even if I could I wouldn't be able to see him. But jeez wish I could.*

Linda F: *Hope Max continues to amaze u with his recovery. Send him our love and also best wishes from friends of ours. Plus, the neighbours are all wishing him well. And as you say, thanks to the wonderful donor.*

Linda G: *What wonderful news, everything has gone perfect. There is a God. Max is such a lovely man, he deserves a good life which he will now have. And as you say, Thanks to the wonderful donor's family, as you have been thanked when you gave Alan's [my Father] liver. C what goes around, comes around. Take care my friend. All is well.*

Linda F: *So happy to hear Max breathing by himself and talking to you- that's more than we could have wished 4 so soon. As u say bless his new heart and God Bless the caring donor's family. What a generous gift they have given. Thanks so much for keeping us informed. Have been all of a wobble all day awaiting this great news.*

Jan: *Oh June. Just read your text and cried. What a relief. Clever, clever surgeons, brave Max and wot a mum he has. Thanks for keeping us updated. Keep textin please.*

Gina: *Just had a little cry for Max, God love him. So pleased the op went well. June we have all been thinking about him. He has so much love and such a dear wife and child and mother! The Best! Xx & Hugs to Max and to you all.*

Reggie: *Well Done. Have all said prayers.*

Pats: *What absolutely wonderful, wonderful news, bless him. Been thinking of you all morning, praying n praying that God will look after him. I cud cry so.*

Mal: *Bless him, he will get thru it, I knew it. That's what mum would have said. My prayers are still with him.*

Jane: *What a relief you must all be so relieved. I'm sending you all so much love it hurts – Now the real work begins. Onward and upwards. Bless you all. Much love Jane x'*

Day 21 – 23/05/10

Had wonderful time with Emma. When she arrived she started crying – no surprise there. She cuddled all of us and couldn't believe how much Alex has changed and how much I haven't!

I took my top off to show her my chest. She was really taken aback. She had seen the picture of me in ICU that mum took (which is glued in) however, all you can really see are bandages and wires and tubes. There was little of my chest in the photo. I said to her that this is nothing. I said my I.C.D bruising was much darker and much bigger and my scar was much more scabby, with a wide fissure at the bottom that was gunky. My chest-drain exit sites were slightly weepy and my central neck line site looked like I had a tennis ball wedged under my skin – which has since completely gone down.

And all of this is to do with the reason I so wanted Emma to come up soon, because she's already missed so much of the empirical evidence of heart transplantation. I fear in another week or so, the sternum scar will be the only thing left to show of what's happened up here.

The chest drain sites and zipper scar will be with me for life, however the sting and abrasiveness of their presence and potency are fading day-by-day. The visual power and intrusiveness of what my body has gone through is very important to me, as you can tell by all the writing in this journal – and anything and everything that is important to me, I want to share with my family.

Tom saw me on that Sunday, which I'm so pleased about, especially because that was one of my bad days. [*On Sunday 09/05/2010 Tom drove up to see me in Ward 27A and then drove back home on the same day. Usually you are only allowed to see the same two people during the first 7 day's isolation period after transplantation. However, as Mum was back home because of Emma's wedding on the Friday (she came back up on the Tuesday), the hospital let Tom visit, just for an afternoon*] Mum and Pam have been here virtually all of the time, so they're a given. However as strange as it seems, am so pleased that Tom saw me in some of my worst moments. He saw the pain, the struggle, the fear, the desperate state I was in. He saw that first hand – with his own eyes and ears and presence – what was happening up here.

You see calling and hearing of events and happenings, even in the most fastidious of details, or seeing photos, or brief video clips (not that we've taken any video clips of anything), or even reading this journal in depth, would just not suffice in providing you with a true idea of what has actually happened here. Whatever knowledge, or understanding, or appreciation phone-calls and photos and Journal reading could give you of what it's been like up here – fresh from heart transplantation – would be of insignificant compare, to the knowledge and understanding and appreciation of actually BEING HERE; like me, like mum, like Pam ... like Tom.

And Tom was only with me for a handful of hours, but in that short time he learnt what it was 'like', much more than anyone at home. And I suppose ultimately, that is what I disliked the most about not seeing Emma and Louise for so long after surgery and my isolation period. I mean Emma rushed up this weekend, but really – it was sort of too late. Louise, I am sure, will be definitely too late – goodness knows how normal my body will be next Saturday with the pacing wires out, the two stitches at the top of my sternum scar removed and my wounds eased after another week of miraculous healing. I mean Emma and Louise didn't even get to see me as an inpatient after cardiac transplantation.

Please, please, please believe me that all of what I am writing is exclusively and solely about my disappointment that I was unable to share what Tom and Mum and Pam have seen and know, with Emma and Louise. I would have loved to have shared that with them, because I am so, so desperately close to them – and they me. That's why I am so gutted I suppose. I am. I admit it. I'm gutted I couldn't share those hard times fully with them. The reasons I couldn't share this with them were, unbreachable isolation, Lou being a teacher, Legsy not allowed time off work, Em's wedding and honeymoon, the logistics of the journey – which altogether made Em and Lou visiting immediately after surgery and isolation, impossible. I bear no disdain or resentment at all, in any way, shape or form to Lou and Em for not coming up – really it was an impossibility. But nevertheless, the disappointment and sadness I feel at their absence is unassuaged by the reason for their absence – no matter how impossible the situation. And I suppose this sadness is spawned solely by the love – the deep sibling love – I have for those two remarkable twin sisters of mine.

Oh it was just magic seeing Emma – it really was. It will be the same when Lou arrives. Man I long for her. Seems so, so long still until I get to be held by her. Patience Max. All in good time.

It seemed we crammed so much into the short amount of time Em was with us for. She arrived at 1pm yesterday and we said goodbye to her today at the train station at 12:20pm. Almost exactly 24 hours!

When Em arrived we meeted and greeted and sat in the garden awhile whilst we ate some lovely French stick rolls that Mum had made. Then, me and Emma only, went for a lovely long walk all through Paddy Freeman's Park, the labyrinth of walkways and paths down the ravine to the forest floor and eventually across to Jesmond Dene and the waterfall.

The weather and scenery and company were just perfect. I just rambled at Emma about loads: de-nerved heart and the delayed normal heart rate response, my anti-rejection medication, Dr Hasan and the Paediatric Team, what it's like having chest drains out (Awful!) and a little bit about those worst days for me – Wednesday to Wednesday in Ward 27A.

She was listening intently, asking lots of questions and really taking it all in. Then we both breezed up that same incline again, continued to circuit the large field of the park and then circled round – back to the lake where we got a drink and I sneaked in an ice-cream! Was lovely. Weather was so hot; too hot. 26/27 degrees in the sun – madness. We were quite literally, on holiday!

We then cruised back and after chilling out for a bit me, Mum and Emma cruised over to the Italian deli, 'Dean and Daniella's' for a wine and a Dandelion & Burdock (an excellent drink!) We sat outside. That was lovely too.

Then that evening we had a wonderful barbeque: proper burgers, sausages, real quality rib-eye steak in Hoi-sin marinade – which was expertly cooked by me I might add – chicken drumsticks, ribs, salad, beetroot and Pam's special potato wedges. Was surprised how much we all ate. And yep, you guessed it again, I ate like a horse!

Watched a bit of Dogma in the evening, however I don't think Em or Mum were into it much – they gave it a good go to be fair – but we shut it down and just chatted until around 10 PM and then all went to bed.

Woke up this morning and Pam was knackered. Alex caught a cold yesterday. He's got two candlesticks hanging down from his nose permanently – more candlesticks than Liberachi – so he woke lots in the night and Pam ended up sleeping in his room with him. So in the morning she was knackered.

So the plan was me Mum, Em and Alex would walk into

Newcastle, have a drink and a quick shop, then say goodbye to Emma at Central station.

The walk was lovely. Took us about an hour/an hour and a quarter. But we stopped a few times at the market stalls on the iron railway bridge and also for a toilet break. Had a lovely drink in the outside seating area at Pret à Manger – was still swelteringly hot, again 26/27 degrees I guess.

We then saw Emma off at the station at around midday; was such a lovely, perfect visit. It really was. Then me and Mum walked back up to the bus terminal, bought some lunch from M&S food court and got the 38 bus back – arriving back here at about 1.30 PM. Perfect timing as Alex was just starting to get ratty for his lunch.

I bought 3 things whilst I was out; well two actually – the third was a present from Mum and I'm just over-the-moon with all three. First I bought myself a pair of quality-lens sunglasses; my eyes and forehead have, since transplant, become really sensitive to bright lights. Am convinced that monster headache I had on Ward 25 when I didn't sleep all night, was because the main overhead light was glaring away past 11 PM.

And during this recent sunny period, in the evenings, my eyes really sting. So the remedy was a nice pair of sunglasses – something I shouldn't have left to Mum to get me on a trip to Sainsbury's by herself. She come back with this pair of 1980's Rayban, original design, rip-off, bubblegum-machine quality, black, barely plastic excuse of a pair of sunglasses. Not only did they cut out less light than a slightly dusty window, they looked awful! They are definitely going back. Anyway, got this pair of total U.V.A and U.V.B protection, level 3 light-reduction hiking sunglasses. Just normal spectacle-like looking frames; metal and Perspex. They're well cool and as clear as a daisy.

The second item was from the stall on the iron railway bridge. It is a photo – wonderfully artistically taken of the Jesmond Dene Waterfall. It's mounted with very thick cream trim and just needs to be framed. It is lovely and so meaningful.

Will frame it and put it up at home so I'm reminded everyday of the miracle that has happened – and the wonderful setting it was all played out under. Of course, how could I forget anyway. But it's the perfect, symbolic abstraction to place in our real home, back down south.

The third is the book that the wonderful Anaesthetist Tim, told us to read: 'Every Second Counts'. It is a book about the circumstances, race and pioneers of the first human heart transplant. In medical ideology, the greatest achievement of the 21st Century. Started reading it when I got home and am completely enthralled and captivated by it. The lead pioneers – like any pioneer I suppose – just have a quest, a mission, it seems, that must be pursued, no matter what the cost.

How mad to have such a calling, such a purpose, such a life mission. Am almost halfway through it already.

Made my lovely prawn, pancetta and leek risotto for me and Pam for dinner. Mmmmn – nice.

WEEK **9**

Day 22 – 24/05/10

Had wonderful time over the hospital, even though I had no appointment over there. Check me out, I'm getting hooked to that place – I really am. It's unlike any other hospital I've been in. The place just resonates a tranquillity, care, love and I suppose beauty – in so many forms. Like the four-year-old, gorgeous little girl I met today in the corridor, with her foster parents and Debbie and Amanda. This little girl was charging around everywhere. She had a heart transplant at one years old, but she also has had other problems. She's had a stroke, so she has a certain (varied and parts unknown due to her age) brain damage – but you wouldn't really know it.

The foster parents, the irrepressible little live-wire girl and Debbie and Amanda radiated such warmth. She is an outpatient – just in for a check-up. When they said to her I'd had a heart transplant too, the little girl pulled the neck on her top down a little to show me her scar. She then pointed to me and I did the same. She smiled and then sprinted off at a hundred miles an hour with her dad hot on her heels, catching her just before she disappeared into the Cardiothoracic Pre-Admissions Ward. Adorable! She still has a long road ahead and will always have problems, but she doesn't know it – not yet anyhow. And so her joy at running around is still just as pure and untainted by the exclusive adult condition of fear for one's own mortality and health. I was with all of them for a good ten minutes. She was such a spirit!!

Well, the reason I was at the Freeman was to play the piano and also because Asif and Amanda have said, on two separate occasions, that I should be around on the 24th. Turns out today is a major Government visit. Due to the baby congenital heart deaths at Bristol ten years ago and other events, it was decided that the best, safest and most efficient way to manage and practice paediatric congenital heart units, is to consolidate the centres around the UK into just a few, large centres.

Basically it boils down to the fact that either Leeds or the Freeman will be closed and the one left open would become the main, larger centre. The idea – Amanda and Debbie said, is considered by most as a good idea, but I can't believe the Freeman Paediatric heart service may be moved to Leeds. Amanda and Debbie said that with the Government and the NHS, you can never be sure of anything. However there would be huge uproar and surprise if it was to be the Freeman that closed. It's even probable that the Government couldn't really do it even if they wanted too. And it's all to do with Dr Hasan. The Freeman has the best transplant record out of all heart transplant hospitals around the world. And that's only since Dr Hasan has been there.

All adult congenital heart transplants are carried out at the Freeman. No-one else will attempt them because they are too hard, but Dr Hasan has the skill and more importantly the will. And apparently, Dr Hasan can carry out surgeries that no-one else will. Basically I get the feeling that if the Government said we want to relocate you all to Leeds and Dr Hasan simply said, 'I'm not going to Leeds', then what could they do? Dr Hasan gets offers for Head Cardiac Surgery posts from all over the world, all of the time apparently – so really, Congenital Heart Surgery cannot lose Dr Hasan. So if he wants to stay at the

Freeman, then I can't see what the Government Board could do. To be honest I don't think they are too worried. Not to mention it's only G.O.S.H and the Freeman who can complete paediatric heart transplantations.

Well I wanted to play the piano anyways, so called Amanda to say I'd be in the Chapel in case I was needed to meet any of the Government representatives – just on the off-chance I was needed to be shown off, so to speak, as a Freeman success story. Turns out I wasn't needed, however Amanda and Debbie came into the chapel to listen to me play and we talked for about half an hour – it was really nice.

The Freeman is also the only place that does the V.A.Ds to an efficiency that lets people be discharged home. They would never close the Freeman Paediatric Unit – am certain. Debbie is a Scouser so whacked out a bit of The Beatles and she loved it … I think!

Also, this morning at about 6 AM, when Pam got up with Alex to get his bottle, she came over all faint and had to lay flat down on the kitchen floor with Alex so as not to pass out. She called out to me to get Mum because I can't pick Alex up yet. She just stayed laying flat for 5/10 minutes. She and me weren't too worried. She knows her thyroid is out of whack what with becoming pregnant and this – along with her hair falling out, were the same symptoms as before. So hopefully she just needs it correcting.

The G.P she saw on Thursday did a blood test and then was going to call the Consultant Pam's under at our local hospital with the results, to confirm what to do. However this all takes time apparently; Pam phoned Basildon Hospital herself and the consultant is away until midweek – all the while her symptoms are getting worse.

Anyways I told Amanda and she instantly said they have a really good thyroid consultant who works with them and he'd be happy to see her straight away. So nice and so helpful. The Freeman and more importantly its staff are just a wonder. So Pam's going to call tomorrow. The blood test that she had at the

G.P Surgery was sent to the Freeman Path-Lab, anyhow. So hopefully Pam will get seen tomorrow. We're not worried though, it's just something that needs sorting.

Then bumped into Carol and Jo (Jo's a 30-odd year old from Southampton who cannot get transplanted because she has 95% antibodies). She was getting her hair cut at the hospital barbers; they are such wonderful people. I talked to the mum Carol whilst Jo had her cut. Was telling her how calm me and Pam were when we knew there was a suitable donor! She was really listening.

Then went David Lloyd Gym for the first time. Done some bike and treadmill. Started jogging for the first time. Was a wonderful feeling, but because hands and toes are really cramping of late, – and when you jog you really grip the floor quicker and tighter with your feet – after one and a half minutes I had to stop, due to the cramping pains in my feet – but my body and legs felt invincible, even for one and a half minutes. Such Freedom. I can't wait until my cramps go. May have had something to do with the long walk yesterday to Newcastle? Or maybe not.

Ooo it's around 7 PM and Mum has just made a lovely chicken and vegetable pasta bake with garlic bread and coleslaw and just before we started to eat, we got a message from Tom to say that Liza is being induced now!!! His phone is off so can't, as yet get any further details, however Liza has made it to just shy of 37 weeks and her liver condition (Cholestasis) has only just come back, so that's probably why they are inducing her now. Don't know anything yet, however it's a far cry from her being rushed to labour at only 31weeks with James. I'll keep you updated, night xxx

Ooo me, Mum and Pam are having a £1 sweep on the weight and sex and date. Bets are:

Mum	5lb6	Girl	Born 25/05/10
Max	6lb	Boy	Born 24/05/10
Pam	5lb8	Girl	Born 25/05/10

Day 24 – 26/05/10 (Morning)

Yesterday was a bad day.

Not about me this time. The transplant journal, this, is all about me and my affairs and thoughts, as you would expect. However yesterday, tragically – not sure yet if the word tragic-ally is appropriate, but it probably is either way – was not about me and heart transplantation.

The facts I know this morning are: Liza was steadily being induced in the early hours of yesterday. It is a slow process, so Tom went home to get some sleep. Liza was then checked at 5 AM and the baby's heart-rate had dropped enough for them to intervene with an emergency Caesarean-Section.

Tom rushed back to the hospital, but was not with Liza in those minutes when she was rushed to theatre for the Caesarean. When the baby was born he was not breathing, or responding. He was immediately rushed to the paediatric High Dependency Unit (H.D.U). Not too long after, little baby-boy Jack Crompton, weighing 5lb8, was taken by ambulance to the Royal London Hospital. Just before he went the staff, as a real exception apparently, wheeled Liza in her bed, with her drips, all the way over to H.D.U – as she was still in recovery herself – to see little baby Jack before he was taken. She didn't, couldn't hold him. Tom followed Jack to The Royal London – Emma rushed there to be with him and Sarah – Liza 's sister – stayed with her.

This morning from what I've understood, the situation is this: Jack cannot breathe for himself, although he is 'rasping' and trying to breathe a little. The doctors suspect, or are sure that it's brain damage. And the extent and severity of the brain damage will be ascertained within the next few days. However the doctor said that the first function of the brain is to tell the body to breathe and at the moment, that's not happening properly. So over the next few days they are going to induce mild hypothermia, to slow and ease the body/brains processes, making it easier for Jack to start breathing. They will then continue to try and reduce his ventilation, to see if Jack's breathing improves. At this point however, I've been told that it doesn't look good.

Apparently Liza is being taken by ambulance this morning to the Royal London, so she and Tom can be with Jack. Yesterday Tom spent hour after hour talking to Jack – who apparently looks like the perfect adorable baby they wanted. Tom says he thinks that talking to him is really helping Jack. He didn't want Emma, who was in the waiting room all day at the hospital to go in and see him – not until Liza was there with them today.

Last night Tom came back to spend the night with Liza in her hospital cubicle – Basildon Hospital specifically put another bed in the room for him. Just as he was going to leave London to go back to Basildon, Tom said that he didn't want to leave Jack. Mum, yesterday, when all this happened, caught the 3 PM train home to be there with Tom and Liza – they need her much more than me now.

This morning Mum drove Tom at 5:30 AM to the Royal London and then was going back to Basildon to be with Liza whilst Sarah has James – not sure what time this morning Liza will be taken up to London, but Tom couldn't wait for that, so he got there early and will be joined by Liza soon hopefully. All the while Jack is in his incubator; ventilated.

There are so many questions, but as we know diagnosis, prognosis and what happened and why, are things that take time. So I will have many more updates as I learn them, however if Jack has brain damage deep enough to not be able to self-respirate, then there can be only one outcome. And that is a terrible, terrible thought. And even if that isn't the case your mind painfully, woefully flutters at the consequences of brain damage and the life Jack may have.

And to think of James, their first-born's struggle at birth:

Born at 31 weeks, incubated and hospitalised for 5 weeks and having Hemiplegia – mildly however, but nonetheless he still has it – again due to a bleed in the brain in-vitro. How can this happen to my brother and his wife and their family? How can it be?

Liza has never been able to hold her newborn baby. Neither has Tom. Liza was so scared throughout her pregnancy about being premature again, that when she got to around 35 weeks pregnant she was so pleased. She was just shy of 37 weeks when she was induced. She had made it – practic-ally full-term. And look what's happened. It's so cruel. So very, very cruel.

A situation like this, I don't even know what to wish for. I've decided to hope for the best for Jack – whatever the 'best' may be. And I hope for Tom and Liza to be with Jack, together, as soon as possible. What tragic wishes aye? It shouldn't be like this. They shouldn't have this happen to them. But it has. And we, them, Jack, will prevail. Nothing is for nothing.

Good luck today Jack. You are in my thoughts and my prayers. Take your time. And do whatever you need. And we'll both trust in the process and keep calm baby ... that's all I can say. Oh and although I haven't seen or met you, I love you dearly.

* * *

As for me, yesterday I had another outpatient's appointment, biopsy, my pacing wires out and was introduced to Jason; a 39 year old from Kent who has been admitted on the Urgent list for congenital heart transplantation. He went to G.O.S.H until he was 18, then The Heart Hospital and now Newcastle. Same path as me. He's on C.C.U (Critical Care Unit) as he's not too well and also has antibodies, so his wait will probably be longer. He was really nice and will continue to pop in to see him.

Have to phone at 1.30 PM for blood and biopsy results so fingers crossed. Just about to go for a walk/jog over the park. Oh and have been started on a new tablet. It's an anti-cholesterol tablet, but Dr Gareth Parry – main outpatient Dr – said it's a tiny dose which has nothing to do with my cholesterol. They have learnt in the last 10 years that being on a small dose of statin (a type of anti-cholesterol tablet) reduces the risk of chronic rejection – the rejection that cannot be cured. So I will lap them up!

5 PM...
Well the jogging wasn't too great. Calves started burning really quickly so I didn't run far, but ran, then walked, then ran again 3 times and as my heart sped up, the distances became slightly longer; only a hundred or so meters, maybe a little more.

After another wonderful waterfall ascent I went over the hospital to see Bobby – he's back up from Kent to sign the transplant consent form and to meet Dr Hasan. Spent over an hour with him and his mum. They were obviously pleased to see me looking so well, so soon. Bob asked me lots of questions about being on the list, getting called and stuff like that. Was nice to share it all with someone in the same boat as me, but just a little further up the river. He will be sent home and then admitted to the Freeman when required.

Later in the day I got outpatient's and 3rd biopsy results. I am showing zero rejection, two anti-rejection medications have been decreased and next biopsy and outpatients is for Tuesday, next week. Have also got to have a blood test this Friday as well. It is really good news, however unlike the last two biopsy results, where I was ecstatic, today I am moderately subdued.

I cannot be happy. Happy really is an emotion I'm not going to find today. Little Jack is still ventilated with no improvement. Details are sketchy as am only getting odd texts from Mum, however earlier in the day Jack deteriorated – don't know the nature of the deterioration – however the doctors managed to stabilise whatever it was, so he's back to normal, in the most tragic sense of the word.

At the moment I see no up side. Sister-Lou asked Tom this morning 'are you hopeful?' He said he's the parent, so he naturally is, however he doesn't think the doctors are. In my mind at the moment little Jack lies on the brink of death. At least now Tom and Liza are with Jack at the hospital.

In the end the transport for Liza would have taken too long, so to get her to the hospital sooner, Louise's Matt drove Mum and Liza there, whereby Liza was admitted to a ward; she still needs hospital attention and treatment following her Caesarean-section. But she'll get that with her new baby son now.

Don't think Tom or Liza have been able to hold Jack. They are just sitting next to his incubator, both talking with him. Tom said to Sister-Lou that when you touch him he does respond, although again details are so limited I do not know the nature of the response – so maybe things could get better? I just don't know. But either way that healthy, bouncing baby they – indeed everyone hopes for – has gone. And it breaks my heart. It really does.

How can I smile at zero rejection when other loved ones are going through such pain, such suffering – such peril. How can my daily transplant successes content me when my new nephew's life is so dramatically and so early in the balance. I just want to cry and cry and cry; for Tom, Liza, James, little Jack and the hardship and torture they have to endure, for the second time.

James' life at Jack's age was also in the balance. How can lightening strike twice, in the exact same spot, to the exact same family? So many thoughts are running through my mind, all of which are premature to think ... the bedroom Tom and Liza painted for Jack, the clothes and presents, Liza 's breast milk, the bigger car they bought for the larger family they should have – organ donation and if so would the heart, if donated, go to G.O.S.H or here? Would Dr Hasan be the Surgeon to transplant it? The Funeral ... when would it be?

Could I go? Major disability and a very poor, very restricted quality of life ... and so, so, so many more thoughts.

But we don't know anything for certain yet. So all these awful thoughts will have to wait. I am just so sorry for them. They deserve so much better.

9.38 PM...
Just spoke to Sister-Lou for 30 minutes. She told me everything which Mum had told her about today. Maybe the worst 30 minute phone-call I have ever listened to. Mum dropped Tom at the Royal London Hospital and then went back to Liza at Basildon Hospital. As Mum walked in at about 7 AM the ward nurse said that it wasn't visiting hours. Mum, it sounds like, steam-rolled over that saying to the Nurse, 'her Husband wants me with her...' Oh it hardly needs any justification does it, but fucking visiting-hour rules – makes me scream.

Anyway she was allowed in. Liza was in her own room, sitting up in bed, knees hitched up, all quiet. She just kept saying to Mum, 'What are we going to do June? What are we going to do?'

Then the transport never happened. It seems like Basildon and The Royal London Hospitals had no idea what they were doing with regards to Liza. They said it would be quicker if they discharged Liza for Mum to then drive her to The Royal London, to then be readmitted there. But this put huge pressure on Mum.

She drove home to get the Tom-Tom Sat-Nav from Matt, then drove back to Basildon Hospital, then parked – which took ages – then realised when getting to Liza that she couldn't walk and needed a wheelchair. So Mum had to go and get the car from the car-parking spot she found right at the other-side of the Hospital, and bring it back round to the front by the entrance.

It was about this time that Tom phoned to say that Jack was deteriorating, so a sense of urgency descended the situation. Mum knew it would be hard for her to drive up to London, park, help Liza out and so on, so Matt came to the rescue. One of Matt's qualities, which I so admire and which reminds me of Dad so much, is that he just 'does'. No fuss, no questions. He just helps, does stuff and doesn't falter in any way.

So Mum pulled up at Matt and Sister-Lou's house (Louise was at school, working), then Matt helped Liza out of Mum's car, into his and with the new urgency of everything, just raced them straight to the front door of The Royal London Hospital.

In the car Liza was just rambling about lots of stuff . . . wanting to be able to give Tom more children, the possibility of a funeral, all the clothes and stuff they'd prepared. She said, 'What are we going to tell people June? What am I going to say?' She also said, 'I don't know if I can see him because I'm scared to bond to him.'

It's important to remember that just over 24 hours ago Liza underwent major invasive surgery under general (not local) anaesthetic. She's on morphine and has had no sleep at all. She was forgetful a few times apparently, which can be the immediate side-effects of general anaesthetic; she thought a few times that she was still pregnant and didn't realise what had happened.

Anyway, at the hospital there was no one there to greet them; no one even at reception. The Royal London is apparently an old, decrepit, tiny, windy, unordered maze of a hospital. Mum and Liza struggled through corridors and around until they found Tom and the Paediatric High Dependency Unit (H.D.U). Liza had all her hospital paperwork and tablets and needed admitting, but the midwife in H.D.U didn't even know who she was when she went in with Tom.

And throughout the day, Tom was meant to be staying in the residential hospital accommodation, but there was even confusion with that. He thought he had a room, then not, then yes. Then Liza thought she could stay with Tom in the accommodation, but once the midwife was brought up to speed she said no way; Liza needs hospital care still because of the bleed risks. So do you know where they put her? On a ward, in a bay, with new mums and their newborn babies! Can you believe it?

So Mum was again in the waiting room whilst Liza and Tom were finally with Jack. Tom just couldn't stop touching him and talking to him. It broke my heart when Sister-Lou, on the phone, told me what Tom kept saying ... 'That's it Jack, well done, you're doing well, that's it, well done, go on, you can do it Jack, you're doing good...' Not a direct quote but you get the meaning.

Mum couldn't even find the canteen, or hot-drink's machine. After a while the midwife asked Mum if she wanted a cup of tea. Mum could have fainted with joy I reckon when the nurse came out with a huge mug, full of tea.

Then getting Liza to her ward was a struggle because she couldn't walk that far and Mum had to hunt down a porter with a wheelchair – sounds madness. Then at the ward Liza and Mum were worried about Tom. Worried about how hopeful he seemed and how much he was encouraging Jack – and himself – to be able to 'get better'; a phrase I am using, not what Mum and Liza said. They were worried that he wasn't attaching to the severity of the situation. But when they asked him he said of course he knows how bad the situation is, but what else can he do other than be hopeful? What else is there left for him to be, other than that? He is fully grounded. As always with Tom, probably more than most.

Anyway that's about it for what happened today. Tomorrow is the third day and if there continues to be no improvement, I think they will withdraw and turn the ventilator off. But that's tomorrow's battle. For tonight I just can't believe what Tom and Liza and Mum have gone through today. Hearing it over-the-phone makes me think that they have been pushed to, surely, the very limit, the very edge, the very cusp of human tribulation. It seems they have been physically, mentally and practically torn apart and fractured and splintered and pounded by today.

I so, so feel for them. I feel so cut-off from them. I haven't spoken to either of them yet. I just want to cuddle Tom, put my arms around Liza and peek, just for a second, at Jack. Oh it's awful. At present my transplant seems to have paled into insignificance. There is a tragedy coming to our family; it's already here and I'm stuck in Newcastle. Away from my family. I wish I could be with them.

Funny how things can turn around. A couple of weeks ago it was Tom wishing he was here.

Life. What is your nature? I just don't know anymore – hell I never did. But now it's even more unbelievable. When will we all be let be for a while? I suppose I'll end today with part of a text I sent to Tom and Liza. . .

Tonight I'm wishing that all four of your family have a peaceful night. It's a tall wish considering the millions of things that must be rushing through your heads, but nonetheless, tonight that's what I'm wishing for. Goodnight Tom, Liza, James and Baby-Jack. Sleep well. Night -x-

Day 25 – 27/05/2010

Spoke to Em and Mum this morning. Mum was telling me just how desperately sad it is down there. How sad it is to see Liza and Tom, entwined in such sorrow, such utter misery. She said witnessing their grief is enough to defeat your spirit, let alone having your own sadness for everything as well. And Mum said that most probably, the worst has yet to come. Oh it's just awful.

Em said she spoke to Tom this morning. He called to ask her to text the Monkey Mums (Liza's baby group) and let them know what has happened, because the last they knew Liza was being induced today, so she had this morning started to get 'well-wishing' texts on the birth – how tragic does this all sound?

Em said she was conscious, as Mum and Liza were yesterday, of Tom being too hopeful to the point of delusion. So she has not as much questioned – she wouldn't be that insensitive and brash – but she sought to qualify what Tom was telling her. Tom said that Jack went a wee in the night which was really good news. Em said, 'Oh does that mean it shows more brain activity?' Tom said he didn't know, no-one had told him that, but that it must be good. Then he said that his brain activity had picked up a little bit last night – the measure which should be 10 and above had been around 2 and went up to 5 apparently. Again Em had caution in her voice when she asked if the doctor had said that was a good thing – to which Tom replied, 'No, that's just what he himself thinks'. He had previously said that Jack's breathing was getting stronger in a positive sort of mood, but the doctors said that they were only seeing slight, temporary improvement – on average there is no improvement. But then Tom, perhaps sensing Emma's caution said 'look Em, I know it's not good and Jack may well die, but all I can do is look for any good and be hopeful'. Em said just to enjoy the moments with him, because moments are so important.

Mum was crying on the phone when she said what happens when a newborn is withdrawn from life support. They take all wires and drains out and the parents, if they want to, get to hold the baby as they pass away. I doubt that in this whole journal of transplantation, you could read a more desperately sad sentence. If there is pain in these pages about life and transplant, well they don't compare to this story with Jack. And what I can't help but think about is that not too many pages back, I said how hearing about events over the phone gives you just a vague, shadowy outline of what is actually happening. So I'm thinking of the horror of what I have interpreted with the fated knowledge that what I'm feeling is just a fraction, just an echo of the suffering and hardship that is being borne down south by my brother and his family.

But I said to Emma that I trust Tom. I trust Tom not to be led astray by disillusioned hope. I trust Tom to hope and look for good and be as positive as he wants to be, without worrying that he is not connecting to the desperateness of the situation. Tom is an enigma to most, but maybe I understand him more than anyone – and I know, I just know that Tom will do himself and his family proud, and I wouldn't question or qualify anything good he tells me. I trust him.

I have not properly spoken to him, or communicated with him, except once this morning. I text him just saying that I hoped he slept and hazarded a joke. I said 'You know what they say, where there's a will, there's a wee' in light of James' (oops, fraudulent error) Jack's wee. He text back for the first time saying 'Thanks, that really made me laugh'. Was pleased he text me back that. Although humour is the natural companion to tragedy, because in such moments the spirit needs to work as hard as it can and humour, along with love, are amongst its most important fuels – but too much humour, or mis-timed humour can have drastic counter-intended consequences.

I remember the night before my friend Tobin's wedding. All the boys were at The Dogs for his last night of freedom when the Vicar called and said that vital paperwork had not been correctly registered, so they couldn't legally get married in the morning. The mood went deathly silent. Then Eddy said, 'Well at least we get to have another Stag-do,' to which Tobin walked off in tears – so you see what I mean. But Tom appreciated it.

4 PM...
Louise called as she left the hospital; Mum's going to stay up there a little while longer. She said there's no change in Jack. They are going to stop the hypothermia treatment tomorrow at 5 PM and then ... I don't know ... reassess? Re-evaluate, I suppose? So they have another day with him at least – unless circumstances change.

Sister-Lou said that she spent most of the day crying – especially when she went in to see Jack. She said he looks perfect. He looks gorgeous. He looks, other than the wires, a perfect, healthy baby. She said Liza, although very sore and unsteady from surgery, seems to be not that bad. Liza cannot be with Jack for too long before needing to come out, where as Tom gets really annoyed and frustrated at being asked to leave even for an hour whilst the Dr's do their ward rounds.

Liza is thinking much more about the probability that Jack will not make it, whereas Tom – although he knows the same – seems to be focused on him being alive in the present. They probably are a perfect balance for one another; each one pulling the other away from depression or delusion.

But Liza slept well last night and is eating; breakfast and a big salad Sister-Lou made for her, however Tom hasn't really slept in two days and has barely eaten. Mum bought him a few rolls today, but he didn't fancy them. He's not eaten, I don't think, since yesterday lunchtime. What must his body be going through? And Liza 's.

But I do fervently believe that everyone of us, deep down, has an ability to withstand the most awesome of catastrophes. The natural human spirit has a resolve, a tenacity, a sheer, irrepressible, unimpedable doggedness that seems to be able – mostly – to stand firm, resolute and just keep, keep going with the echoing words, 'I refuse to be discouraged' and 'I refuse to be beaten.'

You may be beat many times. Maybe Tom and Liza are, and will be. But this enduring spirit that I know is in Tom and Liza will never, ever – I don't think – be beaten. They will get through this, no doubt. However, it doesn't mean that they will not be badly scarred. It doesn't mean that they are not going to be visiting some of the most darkest places, some of the most bleakest corners of their minds, on this treacherous journey that started with Jack's dropped heart rate.

* * *

It's evening now and am awaiting an update from Mum later.

On the Newcastle front Pam was really helped and sorted out today. She knows that her thyroid is out because her hair has been falling out and she had that nearly-fainting kitchen episode. However the temporary G.P surgery she joined took bloods and said to not change anything. Then, once she realised she was pregnant, they redid her bloods, then lost the results, then found them, then lost them again!

When they re-found the results they were going to call Pam's Basildon-Hospital consultant to seek advice. All the while Pam's been getting more knackered and tired.

When Amanda at the hospital asked how Pam was and I told her, she said that she's really good friends with the Freeman's thyroid consultant. So Pam called Amanda this morning and the thyroid consultant called her back a few hours later; he also had both blood test results in front of him – the one's which the G.P surgery couldn't find!

He told her that she now has an underactive thyroid (not overactive anymore) and that she should stop taking her medicine immediately. He prescribed her completely new medication and said that she needs a blood test every week for him to review and that he will personally look after her.

A few hours later we went to The Freeman, ironically for Pam this time. There Amanda, in the Paediatric Congenital Heart clinic, gave Pam her prescription, took her blood – well Debbie actually took her blood, Amanda's side-kick – and said to go to them to get bloods done every week. No queuing in pathology with the normal punters. All sorted. That hospital and staff are just amazing.

Pam and Alex then left the hospital to go home, but I went to play the piano, then to drop off the PSP to Jason – he hasn't got much company so I'm lending him my 24 series and a few games.

On route I bumped into Dr Hasan. I told him all about that

24 hours, the hill, the new life I'm going to have ... He just quietly smiled. I said that I'm so grateful. He said something like it's nice to make a difference. He's as humble as he is quiet. I said I will see him again before I go home to say bye. It was so nice to see him. I think he really liked it too.

* * *

Got text from Tom at just after 7 PM;

Jack Crompton born 5.30 AM Tuesday 25th May 2010. Passed away in his mother's arms at 6.40 PM Thursday 27th May 2010. Loved relentlessly, will be missed forever. Thanks so much for your support. Talk to you all tomorrow. Love Tom and Liza

Now what am I supposed to write now? What can I say?
Blankness ...
Nothing...
At a text like that, my pen stops. I'm devastated. Me and Pam cuddled on the sofa and both cried. Cried and cried. They are probably the most painful tears I have shed in a long, long time. We both just cuddled and cried.
And I'm so FAR AWAY! Just want to get in the car and drive, non-stop, straight home. For the first time I want, need to be back home; with my brother and my family. I'm so cut off. I yearn just to be there.
Tom ... Liza ... Oh Tom and Liza ... I'm so, so, so sorry.
Then an hour later Tom called. He said he didn't feel like he wanted to talk to anyone, but then decided to call. He sounded broken. For the first time I think in my adult life, my strong, older-brother Tom, sounded frail and vulnerable. He just sounded utterly heart-broken. His voice was so pained, so strained, so weak.

He wanted to know how me and Pam were. I told him about my biopsy and all about Pam and her thyroid saga. Then he said what it was like.

He said in that same painful, sorrowful tone, that they took the ventilator off and wires out and gave Jack to Tom and Liza to cuddle. Tom said he shallowly, wheezely breathed for about 30 minutes. Then, whilst he was in Liza's arms, they both watched him take his last breath.

I asked if he was warm, or still cool from the hypothermia? Tom said he was as warm as a normal baby. He also said that Jack was moving his arms and legs a bit. Tom could barely speak. He just kept saying, 'I'm so gutted. Just so, so gutted. I'm tired.' Tom just hasn't slept. He then said he had to go. I said I loved him and will speak tomorrow, or whenever he wants to talk to me. I'm going to stop writing now for today.

Sleep peacefully Jack. God Bless baby.
Your Uncle Max.
Rest in Peace

Day 26 – 28/05/2010 – 6 AM

Awoke with a splitting headache. Think I've been fiercely squinting in my sleep – something I do when I'm having my most disturbed dreams. I almost expected to awake with it. Pam and Alex are still asleep. I just started to cry when I woke up, so have come downstairs to tell you much more about it, as Mum phoned late last night and shared the full details with me; details of the death and how incredibly bitter-sweet it was, but most overwhelmingly, the almost infinite sadness of it all.

I know no details of exactly when or how they were told, however the decision had been made to withdraw treatment.

Tom, Liza, Sarah and Mum followed Jack into a lovely private room. Jack – still on life-support – was put in a lovely white cot

– not an incubator – and Tom and Liza kept taking it in turn to hold him. The nurse said that they could have as long as they wanted. The staff kept coming in on them and said to call them if they needed anything at all, or any reassurance, or if they were worried about anything.

After about half an hour or so – I'm not too sure about the amount of time – the nurse came in and said we will take the ventilator out whenever Tom and Liza wanted; didn't have to be then, they could have as long as they wanted, she said.

Tom and Liza said in almost unison, 'No, you can turn it off now.' Mum and Sarah were, the whole time, just sitting in the corner, silently observing and supporting. You see once they withdraw life-support, they say that they have no idea how long Jack will carry on for. Could be minutes, could be hours, could even be all night.

So the doctor removed the ventilator and Jack was just Jack; no wires, tubes, oxygen. He just rasped with a funny breathing sound, had his eyes closed all the time and Tom and Liza just held him.

Tom took his top off and laid Jack bare on his chest. Mum said you couldn't tell where Tom's chest hair started and Jack's hair stopped – they were exactly the same.

Tom kept stroking him and kissing him and talking to him, as Jack was slowly dying in their arms. Mum said that Tom was saying, '...you're safe, you're with Mummy and Daddy and we love you so much, we love you so much Jack, that's a good boy Jack, strong boy Jack, you're a strong boy...' Hearing that just cut through me like a knife. It's the, '...you're safe...' that shook me so, so much. I kept thinking about those two words. Thinking and thinking and thinking. And he was safe, wasn't he? Although he was dying, he was safe in Tom's arms, safe in Tom and Liza's love, safe in his death.

I do wonder if there could have been anything more perfect Tom could have said to his passing baby boy, other than, 'you're safe, you're with Mummy and Daddy and we love you very much.' They will become immortal words to me. I'll remember them explicitly for the rest of my life. 'You're safe...' how wonderful.

Mum and Sarah popped out of the room after about 20 minutes, but not before the Chaplain came around. Also the nurses came in and, if the parents wished – which they did – they took a little lock of Jack's hair, a foot and hand print of him and Tom and Liza both had photos together with him.

Then, whilst Mum and Sarah were out, Jack took his last, rasping breath in Liza's arms; just the three of them. The nurse came in and confirmed he had passed away and that they could stay with him, again for as long as they wanted. Mum and Sarah came back in.

Throughout all this time all four of them were crying. Probably not every second, but the tears were constant in that room amongst the four of them. Then, after Jack had passed away, Tom and Liza washed him and cleaned him and dressed him in this little baby grow they had and put him back in the lovely white cot.

Tom said to Mum and Sarah that they could hold and touch him if they wanted. Mum stroked and kissed him. The nurse then wrapped Jack in a nice, white sheet and said that when they take him to the little baby morgue, they put a sheet over him so no one else can see him. And Tom and Liza could still visit him anytime for the rest of the day, or night.

But Liza said she needed to be at home. They said their last goodbyes to Jack and then they left. Liza's friend Nat had driven up to the hospital, because she just really wanted to help in some way. She drove Tom and Liza home.

Mum and Sarah got the train to Upminster to get James from Auntie-Iris' and then Sarah was going to have James that night, so Tom and Liza could recover at home and maybe sleep?

Tom hasn't slept properly since Monday. Mum said that she has never before seen Tom shine so much. She said that he gave every part of himself, every possible thing he could give to Jack.

It's like – and these are my thoughts – he crammed years of loving and fatherly care into those 3 days with him. You see the outlook was never good. And maybe a lot of people would at least have had some reserve in such a situation, would have held at least something back, because you know death is likely and the more you are attached, the more painful it would be. I suppose it's an aspect of self-preservation. You know the pain will probably come when the seemingly inevitable happens, so to protect yourself a bit, or look after yourself a bit, you hold a bit of yourself back and you do not hope for too much, or be positive for too long, because that exposes yourself even more.

But Tom. Tom had the courage, that many other dads wouldn't – I'm sure – have had, to give every part of himself to Jack, despite the probable outcome – which he always knew, deep down. He exposed every part of himself. He sacrificed every piece of self-preservation for Jack, because he was convinced that it was helping him. And I know it was too.

Tom, for Jack's sake, got as close to him and hoped as fervently and endlessly and vigorously for him as he possibly could. He gave over his heart and soul, knowing that Jack would not be around to give them back. That's why Mum said that she's never seen Tom shine so. I'm not sure if I've ever heard of a father who, in such turmoil, stayed focused, selfless and in everyway possible helped his poor new baby boy in his short life and peaceful death.

Tom, I cannot say how much I love you. You triumphed for Jack and Jack would have felt that – I'm sure of it.

Mum said that being in that room was such a privilege. She said that those moments were, in a certain way, so lovely and so warming and also that it was the saddest thing that she has ever witnessed. She said the sadness was acute … impossible … extreme. And I think I can see what she means.

In our modern world of presumed immortality, we often view death as the end note. The last word. The most significant detail of any fatal tribulation, or illness, or tragedy. But death isn't just an end marker, a last note, a full stop. Death and the journey to death and the way you die is a part of your life – and maybe one of the most important parts there are.

And when you think about death as a journey, as a path that we all have to walk down, how lovely does Jack's sound? Of course it's tragically far too soon, but when you exclusively think about that road, that journey, that inevitable path we all must take, I doubt many would have such a pleasant, warm, embracing and 'safer' journey than Jack's.

Could there be a better way to go . . . warm and secure in your parent's arms, with them kissing and stroking you, in peace, surrounded by love and care and held tightly and safely all the way along that path to the gates to. . . . . .wherever?

It seems that one of the most wonderful things about Jack's life, was his death. And although that sentence, when read in isolation, sounds as damning and tragic as could be – hell it is tragic – but at the same time, one of the most important things in his life – his death – was perfect. And to know Jack had something so perfect and pure makes me feel really good.

Maybe these are only things you can think and appreciate when you've experienced death; like Dad, Nan, Michael, me – kind of, in Journal 1. I truly believe that as these torturous days painfully fade into the past for Tom and Liza, they will both treasure his death.

*   *   *

Obviously this is a Journal and therefore there are no rules as to what I can write about. However I feel I should say this anyhow, that I will not continue to concentrate solely on Jack and more importantly, Tom and Liza's grief and early bereavement days and so on. Am conscious already that what I have written may already be an intrusion, however detailing in the same length as little Jack's life, Tom and Liza's and our early bereavement pain, would just not be right.

I'll still, if I feel so, write about it and Tom and Liza, however it will not be exclusively. I am also conscious that I, at the moment, am doing so, so well and this is my transplant Journal, so it would also be wrong to ignore, or not write about my joys and triumphs and good news, in light of what has happened with little Jack. If anything it's more important then ever to keep the spirit of this wonderful, miraculous transplant and new life I am starting, burning brightly through the ink in these pages. So I suppose for now, it's back to me and back to Newcastle.

Had just a blood test this morning at the hospital and weight and blood-pressure taken, but that's hardly worth mentioning, except ... oh ... I just did – shucks, too late. Wasn't there long, only about 15/20 minutes in outpatient's, then I went and played the piano for a little bit.

Was really upset though because of Jack, so just played two songs; deliberately two songs only, which were both in light of Tom's and my sadness. I played 'I'm Wondering Why?' Over and over and then the song I play which I think is just the nicest, loveliest, most beautifully sounding song that I can play on the piano – I mean I've played it so much – it's 'On My Own', the title-track from the musical, 'Les Miserable'.

Just looked at the cross above the Altar the whole time. I know I'm not religious, although I do believe that there is something to all of this, however religious or not, there is something very deep and comforting and almost healing about sitting in a house of God and looking at that house's most enduring sigil.

After that I had a Full Monty fry-up in the canteen; wasn't that nice – then cruised home. Me, Pam and Alex then went into Newcastle. I was well tired though. We got the bus into town so hadn't walked much at all, however when we were walking around the shops my feet ached like I had been queuing for hours and hours. They were just killing me, almost straight away.

My feet and hands still feel funny though, due to my medication's side-effects. They go really pins-and-needley when in hot or cold water and kind of numb. When getting into the bath I can't test the temperature with my hand, because all I get is this numb tingling. And when I get into the bath my feet and hands just feel well weird. My feet and fingers are also cramping a lot too. Have still got my hand shakes, but not as bad and not as often – as you can tell by me returning to writing with a pen and not pencil. That's because my shakes have improved, due to my Cyclosporin dosage (anti-rejection medication) responsible for the hand tremors, reducing slowly with every blood test. The most I was on in hospital was 600mg a day, but now after phoning for my blood test results at 3 PM today, it has been lowered again to 450mg a day. But the shakes still come and go. You can tell when I'm having a good or bad day with the hand tremors by the amount and legibility of my writing. Today is a good day. Can you tell?

Anyhow bought a pestle and mortar (for crushing my tablets) and another Journal and a few new pens. Am going with the Pilot G-2 black – the pen that started as a substitute but then took over the world!

Tried to buy some speech-to-text software to start computing these Journals – I'm going to print it out in little bits to share with people I've decided. But nowhere sold that kind of software, so will have to buy it over the internet if I can ever get it working!

Got back and then chilled out for the rest of the day. Had bath and spoke to Craig and Vale – haven't spoken to them in ages, so was on the phone, in the bath, for about 1 ½ hours. I was like a shrivelled prune when I got out!

In the evening I finally spoke to Tom and Liza. It was really nice. Tom had spent today registering the birth and death and they have agreed to have a post-mortem, so the funeral will be at least a week on Tuesday/Wednesday because of the bank-holiday. They both sounded good on the phone. They will both get through this, but it's going to be so hard, with pain that can only be known privately to them; alone.

Then Alex, who's not that well – he's got a chesty cough – was, for the first time, projectile sick; a whole bottle of milk and dinner. Couldn't believe how much there was. It covered the sofa, Pam, him, the carpet, everywhere! Was worried because it was coming out of his mouth and nose and momentarily he couldn't breathe. But he was okay and slept through the night – as usual.

Well that's it for the 28/05/2010 and this second Journal. See you in Journal 3.

Bye -x-

Journal Three

Day 27 – 29/05/10

New journal, but unlike the start of my second journal, 'not' the same heart! Wow. I still can't believe it all. I really can't. Do I really have a 35 year old stranger's heart in my chest? Do I? Well yes and it's a privilege too, nonetheless. I still haven't contemplated my donor, Andrew, much. I have tried, but I get distracted by everything else that's been happening. And lets face it, there's been quite a bit. I suspect I will really ponder Andrew, his fate, his family, his tragic loss later – when the winds and noise of Newcastle and the onset of my new life, ease to a breeze and a hum. I wont force anything too soon.

Ooo guess what? Sister-Lou and Matt are visiting and should be here at around 1 PM; two and a half hours time. Yay! Matt going back tomorrow, but due to school holidays, Lou is staying until Wednesday. Double Yay! Am just off now to walk Alex to Sainsbury's and back. One, to get him asleep and the other to get some Febreze to spray the sofa, because it smells of sick!

WEEK **10**

Day 29 – 31/05/10

It's Bank Holiday Monday morning and I'm sitting in the living room with little, perfect Alex. It's about 6:45 AM. Have taken Alex downstairs so Pam can carry on sleeping. She's been so tired bless her. The early pregnancy tiredness is really starting to hit her and her unbalanced thyroid is probably not helping much either. So Alex is just sitting on the floor – his doughnut play-ring in front of him packed full of all his toys; big ones, bright ones, noisy ones, flashing ones, small ones and all sorts and right now he is playing with the sofa cushion I put on the floor, to break his fall if he falls back.

I tell you as I'm writing he is pulling the pillow this way and that and when I look up at him, he dunks his head down onto the pillow and just beams his adorable, pearly-white smile straight at me. I tell you Alex is just so gorgeous. And he's growing and learning oh so much. He really responds decisively now and is more knowing by the day. I played the first fully interactive, reciprocal game with him a few days ago. It was such a lovely moment. It was the first time I've played with Alex and he has actively played back, actually instigating and leading the game. I was getting him dressed on our bed. He was just in his nappy so I started to play my 'chuck away' game – what Emma used to do with baby Ben I think. Literally you just fling

Alex over from back to front so he bounces on the bed and gets thrown about a bit. He absolutely loves it and laughs so loud . . .

Ooops, Alex has just fallen back and whacked his head on the floor in the only spot that I didn't cover with a pillow! No tears though, which is a surprise. I've just sat him back up again and he is busy playing with a broken Sky remote control that we have given him, so he stops trying to get ours.

Anyway, on the bed the 'chuck away' game developed into me just rolling Alex from his back to his front one way, back onto his back and then rolling him onto his front the other way – like he was a rolling pin going back and forth. He was loving it. Every time he rolled onto his back, facing me, I shouted 'there you are' and he cracked up. Anyhow I decided it was time for me to get him dressed, so left him facing me whilst I reached for his clothes and stuff. Then he, on his own, rolled over, pushing his face flat down on the bed. Then, after a few moments, he'd quickly spring back looking up at me – me saying 'there you are' again. Then he'd do it again and again. As he waited face down I started to voice a 'wooohhh. . . . . .' build up, getting louder and louder and Alex would pause, for longer and longer, until he snapped back onto his back, beaming and laughing. It was so funny, so lovely. The first totally interactive game I have played with him. Of course now as soon as you lay him back to get him dressed he instantly thinks it's rolling-pin time and rolls away. Oops. Still nevermind, aye?

In saying that he's been a right so-and-so this morning. Started grizzling when I was on the previous page so took him into the kitchen, put him in his walker and gave him a chunk of banana to munch on whilst I made his Weetabix. Then he didn't want his Weetabix. Started grizzling. I realised I made the Weetabix with cold milk, so heated it up for him. He still didn't want it. Gave him some water, didn't want that. So plonked him back on the floor, didn't want that. Just wanted to whine. So I just left him on the floor. After a few minutes he gave up on the whining and returned his attention back to the Sky remote! Ahhhh – peace.

But that boy is just so, so perfect. So gorgeous. It's been difficult for me, not being here at night and in the mornings, before transplant. Not being able to read him his books, put him to bed, spend the morning hours with him – some of the best hours of the day with him, if you ask me.

And immediately after transplant I couldn't see him. Then only briefly on the ward, or 27A's kitchen, or outside if the weather was nice. And when I first got home I couldn't hold him at all or get that close to him because of scars, pacing wires, neck-line bruising. But now I can really start to parent Alex again. I can feed him now (my hands are much less shaky), hold him and move him a bit, have him sit with me and read his books, go on walks with him, dress him and other stuff too.

So I have really started to feel in this last week, that I've been making up for some of the lost time and lost things that I have not been able to do with him. And already he is going to me more and favouring me more. It's so nice. That boy is just so wonderful. Too utterly, utterly perfect.... except the whining, which has just started up again.... !

Been having a lovely time so far with Louise and Matt. Saturday we went for a long walk with Alex (Pam rested in bed), through Paddy Freeman's, down to the waterfall, along the river to the iron railway bridge, then back round to the park.

Then me, Matt and Lou went to the lovely Indian restaurant that me and Mum went to, pre-transplant. Was lovely. I ate so much. Much too much mind, my belly was hurting through bloating pains a little later.

Yesterday Matt went for a run and then tried to unblock the two drains out in the garden which he spotted were overflowing a bit. Bless him, he is so helpful and caring. He also offered to mow the front lawn; I use the word lawn in the very loosest sense of the word – mow the front forest would be more befitting. But the weather was on and off and he had to leave at 11 AM anyway.

Me, Lou and Alex walked to Sainsbury's to get lunch – Pam

again rested in bed; she really needs the rest. In the afternoon Lou, Pam and Alex had a sleep and I went over to the Chapel to play the piano. Whilst there I decided to re-word the song Tom wrote and sent to me, 'I'm Wondering Why'. I was in the Chapel for about an hour-and-a-half rewording the three verses. It was all about.... well, obviously the heartbreaking fate of Jack, although I haven't explicitly mentioned it. The lyrics, including the main chorus line which I left unchanged are below:

CH: *I'm wondering why...? Tonight.*
      I'm wondering why...? Tonight.
V1: *Beauty has as many faces as tragedy,*
      And its hard to find just one of them without the other's company.
      The Hell you two have been living through I'm aware I cannot know,
      But sitting at these white keys I'm sure I see beauty too ...
      so I say...
V2: *Life's enigma is so bare when you look and see,*
      The wonder and the pain poured down on this one family.
      Alone now in this Chapel I just feel so far away,
      Cause there's nothing I can say to you I just wanna hold you every day...
      so I say...
V3: *It's hard to find a third verse to this song worded for you,*
      I've tried my best but the first two verses are all that I could do.
      Time ticks on and on and on as it always does,
      And I'm sure that we'll all find our peace deep inside each others love ...
      so I say ...

Later I wrote that out and sent it to Tom and Liza – I'm really pleased I done it.

Lou-lou made a lovely dinner, chicken roast and we all wolfed it down. Well, that brings me to now. Me, Lou and Alex are going to walk to the swimming pool soon – Pam's still resting. She's given so much these last few months, she deserves all the rest she wants!

*   *   *

Well had such a lovely day today. Alex was gazonked in the morning. Just before we left at 10 AM he had his bottle and went asleep, so plugged him in his cot and only me and Lou walked to the pool. The weather was so nice, really, really sunny and really warm in the sun. The walk into the park, down the ravine, across the waterfall, up the other side and into Jesmond to the pool, was really nice.

When Lou was swimming I got a drink from Subway and sat on the outside seats, in the radiant sun, with my excellent sunglasses and read my book 'Every Second Counts'. Nearly at the end of it. Absolutely fascinating. It was such a lovely morning. Then we walked back the same way, as the temperature of the day increased and sat by the lake and had a lovely cup of tea and I had a cheeky strawberry ice-cream. Got back at 12:30 and spent the rest of the early afternoon in the garden, sunbathing, reading and chilling.

Pam was starting to feel better as well so we both walked Alex to Sainsbury's to get a few bits for the Spag-Bol tonight – my turn to cook. Then, on the way back, we stopped at Dean and Daniella's, still drenched in rich sunshine and had, at the outside seating, two dandelion and burdocks and some mixed olives and ciabatta. Was so, so lovely. The ciabatta came with the usual olive oil and balsamic, except it was not balsamic vinegar. It was this heavily reduced balsamic glaze – kind of like sweet balsamic molasses. Was gorgeous. And with the mixed olives, the dandelion and burdock, my family, the sun, my amazing health and recovery and the lovely day, it's hard to imagine how life up here could be going, or could have gone any better.

Spoke to Tom in the evening. He and Liza today planted an Apple tree in their garden in memory of Jack. Apple trees blossom in May. Such a contrast. I wish I could feel what it's like at home at the moment. I've tried and tried to imagine, but I can't and with the sun, the lovely day and the joy up here, it makes connecting to Tom and Liza and the reality of what has happened, all the more impossible. But it's just the way it has to be I suppose.

Biopsy and outpatient review tomorrow – must remember to down a good few glasses of water as soon as I wake up, so I'm not 'dry'; dehydrated. So when Dr Gareth Parry digs around in my neck to find my right subclavian vein, he doesn't have to dig too deep, or for too long, as the more hydrated you are, the higher the veinous pressure and therefore the more plump and prominent the veins are … the power of water!! Drink-drink-drink Max, for your poor neck's sake. Night -x-

Day 31 – 02/06/10

Louise left early at 5:30 AM this morning. I was awake so got up with her and had a quick cup of tea whilst we waited for her taxi; only 10 minutes or so and then she was gone. I just can't tell you what a wonderful time I have had with Lou. I really, really have. And because she was here for a comparatively long time for a visit – Saturday to Wednesday – it was such quality, quality time. I felt like we really connected and bonded in ways that we do not usually. I mean Pam was resting a lot, so for lots of walks, cups of teas out, outpatient check-ups, cooking dinners and so on, it was just me and Lou. Not sure if I've ever spent such an amount of time exclusively with Lou, so close together. It was just wonderful.

Louise has though, like we all do, some habits/personality traits, that can grate on me the wrong way – like the obtuse labelling in Journal 1. But these are such minor infractions.

They really are. Spending this much time with Lou you realise one overriding thing – she just cares for people so, so much. The way she was talking about Tom and Liza, the way she was with me, the way she was with Pam – helping us both so much with Alex and domesticities so that Pam could rest and I could recuperate.

Her heart just pours out love all around her, splashing everywhere, this way and that, a continual flow, a constant torrent of compassion and concern for others. She really is a genuinely loving and giving creature. She's done so much for us here: tidying up, looking after Alex, cooking, cleaning, constantly asking if I wanted a drink, or anything from the kitchen.

Yesterday – after outpatients and biopsy and an hour-and-a-half snooze, which me and Pam had whilst Lou looked after Alex – Me and Lou went on a power walk. Well I'm calling it a power walk anyway. We walked through the park, down the ravine, back up the other side, into Jesmond, past the swimming pool, onto the road back to the Freeman, then – as the road re-crosses the river – we picked another ravine trail, crossed back over the river, up the really steep route back to the park's summit, lapped round Paddy Freeman's again, back to the lake and home in 55 minutes – marching pace the whole time.

Was exhilarating, such a good feeling. Was sweating and breathing heavily, blood coursing through my veins, heart pounding in my chest and eyes, and I could not have felt more alive, vibrant, normal, or proud...♫This new heart of mine ... I'm gonna let it shine ... let it shine ... let it shine ... let it shii-iiiiiiine...♫

*   *   *

Yesterday's biopsy was the best yet. I drank three glasses of water from about 6 AM, so when Gareth went digging around in my neck he hit my right subclavian at the first attempt. The biopsy, which usually takes 20-30 minutes, was over in 9 minutes. And because he only inserted the needle once (no digging around) my neck feels nowhere near as sore as it usually does.

Whilst I was waiting for the Biopsy I got chatting to this guy next to me who was also having one done too. His story was that a couple of years ago he started to be sick a lot. The G.P said something about a type of vertigo? G.Ps!! The sickness got worse, he went to his local hospital and they saw that his liver and kidneys were enlarged. The hospital accused him of being on drugs and wouldn't believe that he wasn't!

Then he went to his General Hospital and they diagnosed him with Cardio-myopathy (a disease that destroys the heart muscle – incurable). He spent a year deteriorating on the heart transplant list. Then, when he only had a week or two left to live, he had a Berlin Heart fitted – an external mechanical heart whereby big tubes of blood, come out of the chest to connect to a big cooler-box sized, noisy machine, which then pumps the blood back into and around the body. He said that the Berlin Heart operation came with a 10% chance of success. 10%!! 90% chance of fatality.

However, in light of how little time he had left, he went for it. He was on the brink of death. The operation was successful and he was sent home with his Berlin Heart – not like the V.A.Ds, not sure if he was allowed out really, more like home-bound, hospital release. Then after 11 months of having this noisy, suitcase-sized machine, with thick tubes of blood connected through his chest (I suppose like having chest drains in all the time) he was called for transplant.

It was his first call and he was only brought in as a reserve – if the doctors are not sure that the patient they want to give the heart to is going to be compatible, they bring in a stand-by at the same time, to ensure that the heart is not wasted. Anyway it was his first call and he was only on stand-by, however due to anti-bodies he was more suitable and was transplanted.

It took him one week to wake up after the surgery. Another

week until he was fully 'with it' and out of I.C.U. But now? He is 6 days away from the most important and significant milestone of heart transplantation – the '1 year out' mark. In 6 day's time he'll be a year out and from then on the risks of so much should go down and it should – only 'should' mind – be plain sailing.

And to add to the success, he – touch wood – has not had a single rejection episode. He's back at work with a perfectly normal life and a few months ago, he married his fiancée. They were due to get married two years ago, not long after he become unwell. So they married in January. I said I bet that was one special wedding. I privately thought of all the cynicism that surrounds weddings nowadays and at how all of that pessimism is such bollocks when you consider the worth and value of their wedding day; it must have been so special – as it should be. He said it really, really was and that how she was a rock for him the whole time. I said the same about Pam.

Then he said how scared he was before the transplant and that when he left his wife at the operating room doors, he said 'see you later'. I asked if he said those exact words. He said yes, they planned it that way. Not sure if I've written in the previous journals or not, but right from the start, when me and Pam knew I was going to someday have a heart transplant, we planned that our last words before she left me for the surgery were going to be – 'see you later'. And they were.

Co-incidence, this guy and his partner decided the same words? And when you think about it, there are no better parting words, before major surgery, other than 'see you later', oh and of course, 'good luck'!!

At outpatients I finally caught up with Lynne – I popped my head into the transplant office. Was good to catch up with her. I said that I would type up my Journal and send a copy into them and she was quite pleased I think – she wont be when she sees the size of it!! As I was chatting to her Dr Hasan came in to talk to one of the other transplant co-ordinators about another case. He said hello and asked if I've got my marching orders yet. He also said, because he seems to see me about so much, that I'm becoming part of the furniture! He's probably right, but at least I had a genuine medical reason to be at the hospital today! Unlike other times when I'm visiting Jason, Bobby, or just playing the piano.

* * *

Am now sitting in the garden. It's a glorious day. Alex is in his pushchair going to sleep – just had his bottle and it is time for his late morning nap. It's about 11 AM. Have the gazebo up, Pam's put the washing out and am just going to relax and chill in the garden until John and Jen turn up around 2-3ish, I think. I can't wait for Pam to see her Dad and sister again – she's so missed them, as they have her. Will be so, so nice. Alex has drifted off now – hopefully that will mean one or two hours of peace and quiet!!

I can't believe I had an Orthotopic Homocardiac Transplantation just over four weeks ago. I just can't believe it. Me and Pam were talking about it last night when we went to bed. We were saying, when you think about it now, how scary it seems when you look back at the 'before transplant' period. If they said that I needed a heart transplant now, I'd be so scared. I'd fall to bits. It would be impossible to imagine. But we done it. We were there and we coped. We talked mainly about the hours preceding the operation – from when Neil came into my room on Ward 30 at 1:30 AM on Monday 3rd May, until we walked out of my room at about 6:20 AM.

You see when I think about those hours now, it's from a new perspective of now being safe; of not really having to potentially face death today. Now I know we all do technically face death every day, but this is a mere technicality – emotionally and perceptually we do not. We – other than the cold secondary whisper of logic, which always comes after your emotive perception of something – do not believe that we face, or indeed could meet death today, tomorrow, next week, or anytime in the near, or even not so near future. We are secure within ourselves. We're safe within ourselves. We are so confident within ourselves, that that secondary whisper of logic fades into almost nothingness – far down into the back waters of your mind, virtually out of reach, so far from daily thought and deed that it really, really is, for all intents and purposes, non-existent.

I suppose it's a product of the world we now live in and the time we now occupy in humanity's journey. We – and I will not go into who 'we' are, I imagine you can tell roughly who I am talking about, most people who live in a modern world like me – are more safer now than at any other point during human history. We are more secure and stable now than ever and therefore why would we get up every morning thinking that we may face death today? I mean in our average, day-to-day lives, what is there to remind us of our own mortality? What is there to show us that we are not indestructible for that day? Nothing. Nothing what-so-ever. I know there are many exceptions to the group 'we' that I have labelled. But the bulk of us, I think, which I hasten to say now includes me, do not believe that we are going to walk today, through The Valley of the Shadow of Death. And maybe this could be seen as one of the triumphs of our modern world – one of the real benefits of the 21st Century, that many of us are protected from the fear of death, day-to-day, month-to-month, year-to-year. Or perhaps you could say it is one of this world's greatest losses – the loss of that daily respect for self-existence, loss of that knowledge of actual mortality.

However that's a different argument that I'll leave to the philosophers. But the point I'm laboriously making is that last night when me and Pam replayed those hours between 1:30 AM and 6:20 AM, we couldn't, from our safe warm bed, believe how calm we were that night.

Now I haven't actually written about those hours yet, so I will briefly say what happened . . .

Neil came in to my room with the ward nurse and said about

the potential donor. The ward nurse gave me a big hug. Then Neil asked if I was okay and how I was feeling. And you know what? I didn't really feel anything. Then, over the next few hours, me and Pam (I called her straight away and she came over) went for a chest x-ray, had bloods taken and had to shower with that special red anti-bacterial, anti-fungal goo. Then I shaved my chest, face, neck and femoral vein area (inside of thigh/groin) with these absolutely stupid razors the hospital gave me – it was ridiculous, but managed it in the end. Spoke to Mum, Tom, Em and sister-Lou. Said I was going down to theatre at 4:30 AM (original estimated time) and that I loved them and would speak to them when I could.

Mum phoned Uncle Dave to immediately drive her up to Newcastle, which had been pre-arranged. Then me and Pam laid on my bed together. I took off Dad's necklace, my wedding ring and my S.O.S bracelet. Pam threaded the ring and bracelet through the necklace and put it on. And we just laid there. Calm, collected, comfortable and peaceful. We were so relaxed Pam even fell asleep.

The operation was delayed so 4:30 came and went, then 5, 5:30, 6.... and still we just snuggled. I cannot tell you how tranquil it was. We were so safe, it felt. So serene, so soft and gentle, so simple. There was no panic, no fretting, no tears even. It was bizarre. I had no idea it would be like that. Then we both walked down to theatre.

At the doors to the clinical operating rooms we both gave each other a little peck on the lips and an almost cursory, customary cuddle – no tight everlasting powerful embrace, no scrunching each other as tight as we could with tears and dread, just a quick cuddle. We both said 'see you later' and we happily smiled and she walked out. Even then my calmness and tranquillity stayed constant; impenetrable.

As I was well and in all other ways healthy, I walked into theatre; transplants are classed as emergency operations, therefore there is no pre-med. Then, as they started putting the cannulas in my right hand and left arm, the hospital phone went. Neil, who was co-ordinating the timings, said the donor's kidney Surgeon was delayed, therefore it would be another 30/40 minutes before they looked to clamp off the donor's heart.

So in the operating theatre, next to a trolley with scalpels and saws and the heart bypass machine, under those impending, menacing, bright surgical umbrella lights, with my ECG, De-Fib and brain activity pads on, they turned the operating table into a chair and me, the really nice paediatric anaesthetist Tim Murphy, the whole operating team and even Dr Hasan, for a little bit, were all just sitting around, chatting. We talked about football – Tim's a big Arsenal supporter – a strange residential disturbance that 'Big Dave' – a 7ft giant of a man on the team – had the previous night and other casual banter.

It was just so surreal, so amicable, so natural, so burdenless. I remained just as calm, just as relaxed, just as at peace with myself and my world and my uncertain fate. I felt safe somehow, despite the danger, despite the uncertainty. I do not know why that was, but Pam said she felt, in those long hours before surgery, just as calm as me.

And when we talked about it in bed last night I realised why. You see ever since we were called up here to live on the transplant list we have, every day, actively, at the forefront of our minds, with every part of our perception and at every ranging emotion known that today I could, really, really could, face death. In fact it was a certainty that I was going to walk through The Valley of the Shadow of Death at any moment – literally at any moment.

It wasn't a cold secondary whisper of logic that made me know it, it was being immersed in the Freeman Hospital. It was being fully, physically entwined with the sounds and smells and realities of living in the Cardiothoracic block of the Hospital. There is nothing like hearing cardiac monitors every night, or exchanging with Pam the parting phrase 'See you tomorrow honeys, or in the middle of the night for a transplant' –

something we said every night – right in your face, unavoidably real, relentlessly reminding me that absolutely any day now I would face death – even if it were a 10% chance of death. You see this is why we were both so calm. For 5 weeks we had been living with that knowledge. For 5 weeks we had known that at any moment I was to undergo major, life-threatening surgery. That's why we were calm. Because we were so ready, so prepared, so equipped and in the end, at peace with the uncertainty we have had in these 5 weeks and to a lesser degree, ever since Fiona Walker said about heart transplantation for the first time back in March 2009.

Finally, after all that time and adjusting and forgoing of usual everyday assurances of safety and immortality, we reached a point, during those hours between Neil's first visit and being put under, of utter acceptance. We had truly surrendered that most basic of concepts that we all think we all hold in our normal, immortal world – CONTROL. We had finally surrendered control and were, to borrow a phrase from Mum, at rest and at peace within a 'safe uncertainty'.

I now realise why we were so calm and that why last night, when we contemplated it afresh, it seemed so invincibly scary and terrifying. It's because now we are starting to look at the whole thing from the pulpit of a new found immortality. And indeed when normal people drop their jaw and say 'I don't know how you coped', or 'I don't know how you did that', or 'I wouldn't have been able to', they are also, just like me and Pam last night, looking at the whole thing from the indestructible integrity of presumed immortality, inherent in our normal day, modern world living.

You see things really aren't as bad when you get down to the same level to look at them. Anyhow being terrified of that whole thing now, shows that Pam and I now feel and believe in a greater certainty in our life – although nothing is ever certain, especially 4 weeks after transplant. However there is already now more certainty, which, considering the unknown we have had to constantly battle with over the last year/year-and-a-half, is just such a RELIEF! A huge ominous weight is slowly but surely lifting. And within that liberation from major-uncertainty's burden, a life-anew is beginning for us. Long, long may it last...

Day 32 – 03/06/10

I didn't tell you about the outpatients/biopsy results. Well they were really good. Biopsy result was minimal. Am going to find out exactly what that means tomorrow. In essence it's as good a result as zero rejection, as biopsies are now fortnightly, YAY! Also outpatients review is now weekly but still need blood test tomorrow. They have also reduced my Cyclosporin from 450mg to 400mg a day. And my hands are getting better all the time.

Not sure if when I've called before and they've said zero rejection, it actually means the same thing as minimal rejection (and different people just say it differently) – maybe? Pam seems to remember when being told about rejection, that there are many different grades/severities. And that you could be minimal which doesn't register as a rejection episode. Either way my appointments and biopsies have stretched out and anti-rejection meds decreased, so the result is, I think, the same as zero rejection. However, as I said, will find out specifically tomorrow – not worth phoning about now. You'll just have to wait on the edge of your seat until tomorrow!

It looks like the funeral for little Jack will be tomorrow week – Friday the 11th. Not certain until the post-mortem is started, however that's the provisional date. I asked Dr Parry about it and he said it would be ok for me to go. However, on that Friday, Pam has her important appointment with the Thyroid Consultant and she can't miss that.

So the plan was going to be that John, after leaving with Jen on Sunday, would come back up on Wednesday/Thursday for another couple of weeks. Also on Wednesday Mum was going to fly up and then me and mum, in my car, were going to drive back home for the funeral the next day. Then either Tom or Eddy were going to, on the Sunday, drive with me back up, because although I can now drive, I wouldn't be able to do the whole journey by myself – so one of them would do it with me, then I would pay for their plane, or train fare home.

You've probably detected the use of the words 'was' and 'would' rather than 'am' and 'will'. That's because Tom phoned me this morning as me and John were walking Alex around the park – again drenched in Louis de Bernieres Kefelonian sunlight. He said he would prefer it if I didn't go to the funeral. I said of course, that's fine, whatever you want. Then he tried to explain, the both of us knowing he wouldn't be able to and that he didn't need to. All he said that was clear enough to draw meaning from was, 'I just wouldn't want it that way'. And I think I know what he means. I'll leave it at that. As I've said before, so much of Tom is an enigma and he is so deep, that so often he struggles to explain himself – probably in the same way that I, even with my best tool, my writing, cannot explain how I understand him either, or necessarily what it is that I understand. Which is why I'll leave any explanation there. But nonetheless, I think I might understand the reasons he cannot say and I cannot write.

I said Tom that's fine, it really is. I said please don't give it another thought. I also said how pleased I am that he himself was able to call me up and tell me directly that he didn't want me to go. He said it wasn't easy for him to do, but not too difficult for him not to do it.

I suppose there isn't much more that could speak higher of the inexplicable bond between two brothers, when one phones the other and says, without fear or guilt, I do not want you to come to my three-day-old, baby boy's funeral. And for such a request to be met with respect, compassion and – and I'm writing as sincerely as I can – without the slightest bit of resentment, frustration or grudge.

It's probably for the best. And I respect Tom's wishes with the utmost understanding and love. I will miss them and the funeral terribly though, but things are never perfect and what a hideous concept perfection is anyhow – maybe one of the greatest evils we face today, through the guise of virtue... But I'll leave that to the philosophers too.

Day 33 – 04/06/10

It's about half one in the afternoon and I am at home all by myself for the first time, I think? Not sure if I mentioned that my work are going to stop paying me in a week or two's time, so want to try to catch up with Tessa, (the transplant team's social worker) to see what stuff I'll be able to get financial help with. Because in a weeks time mine and Pam's joint salary will be £200 a week with a mortgage, a rented property, a baby and one on the way – Yikes! Tighten the belt times, me thinks. Still we have got some savings to use, so we shouldn't be too bad.

Have lots to tell you today, but didn't finish off telling you about yesterday, so here goes:

Had a nice day. Me and John walked Alex round the park in the morning as I've said, then we drove to Waker's River walk – just a path along the Tyne, or Weir, not sure which, into Newcastle. However it was really hot and Alex was getting ratty straight away, so we turned back home for lunch and some shade. Got some fish n chips ... mmmnn. Then just chilled all day in the glorious weather in our lovely little garden.

Had to pop over to the hospital around 3:30 PM for Pam's thyroid blood test. Debbie quickly took it in the Congenital Heart Clinic and also she had typed me a letter I asked for, for work – just a Dr's note really, nothing more, officially stating that I've had a heart transplant so they can arrange my sick pay and statutory sick pay.

Then, guess what, we were slobbing about so much we

couldn't even be bothered to go to the supermarket for dinner, so we got a blow out Pizza Hut. So nice, but what a terribly unhealthy day for food! All four of us, Me, Pam, John and Jen played Nomi again that night and it was, as before, hilarious – so much so that I was considering taking a few Paracetamols before I went to bed – the pain from my surgery when I laugh is just unbearable.

*   *   *

Well today I split from the others. Lynne called me last night to see if I could go and see this girl, similar to me, Jason and Bobby – also in C.C.U awaiting a heart transplant. We also needed to go on an Asda shop for lots of bits ´n bobs and Pam, John and Jen wanted to go into Newcastle. So, as I needed a blood test in the morning, we decided to split. Also it would give Pam some nice time alone with her Dad and sister – oh, and Alex. So they went shopping and then Newcastle; John had his anti-coagulation blood test at the hospital in the morning as well.

I had my bloods done, went gym for a 40 minute workout – which felt really good – went on the internet for a bit and then went over to the hospital to see Jason and Lorraine. Got to the hospital at 10 AM and left at 12:30 PM. Was with Jason for a while and then he introduced me to Lorraine. Lorraine was actually in theatre having a hickman/pick line put in. It's just like a cannula into an artery, however it's long-term, therefore the procedure is more befitting to a catheterisation – burrowing down more, so infection risk is much less and the line can stay in for months.

So I spoke for quite a long time to her mum, Andrea. Lorraine's recent story is just amazing. I have never heard of such a real life – and by 'real life' I mean listening to the mum, and watching the mum, and feeling the story, through her eyes, her watery, welling eyes – I don't mean reading these glossy

'OK' magazines from the comfort of your sofa, with a forlorn, contrived, over dramatised photo of the person or family telling the story.

Four years ago Lorraine felt a few funny heart beats in the evening, which only lasted a little while so she didn't think much about it. The next day she went to see her mum in the library where she works and told her about it. Her mum said are you sure you are ok, perhaps we should tell the hospital? They are from Northern Ireland and they have been going to the main Congenital Heart place – The Royal Victoria, I think, all of Lorraine's life.

Anyway as soon as Andrea said that, Lorraine just collapsed in her arms. She shouted out for help and a First-Aider came over to give Lorraine mouth-to-mouth whilst Andrea compressed her own daughter's chest – she had no training, just doing it from what she'd seen on T.V and stuff.

Opposite the library was a kind of community health centre, which usually just has administrative staff for information purposes only – like a kind of family planning clinic or something like that. There may be the odd district nurse there, but no more. However on that day the place was hosting a training course, so when someone from the library ran over to get help, six doctors came running over – probably the only time there has ever been that many doctors in the centre.

Anyway they started working on Lorraine until the para-medics arrived. The paramedics then worked on her, all the while the Mum was kneeling by her side – pleading with the paramedics to continue. It was only due to the mum asking them to continue treatment that the paramedics shocked her for a second time. But still no response. The doctors started to move away and get people's names and the paramedics stopped and just looked at each other across Lorraine's body and were about to pronounce and confirm death – it was 25 minutes since Lorraine had collapsed.

The mum however, pleaded with them to try defibrillating

her for one last time – her daughter had pretty much died in front of her, in her arms. The paramedics looked at each other again and just as they were deciding what to do, on the floor of the library, with everyone around, Lorraine's heart came back to life. For some reason it just restarted – maybe because of the adrenaline and other meds the paramedics administered, or maybe because God himself said, 'That's enough, you can stay Lorraine'.

And even then the fortune continued as the local hospital she was rushed to was being visited, that day, by one of Lorraine's own specialised Congenital Heart Consultants from the Royal Victoria in Belfast. He was giving a seminar, but was brought over and knew Lorraine's condition and history straight away, so he knew what should and should not be done. Something a hospital would not know due to the complexity and individuality of a rare heart condition and cardiac history.

Lorraine was unwell for a long time and has since never returned to work, but she hasn't lost any brain function – initially she was dazed and not fully 'with it' for quite a while, but after a year or two she was almost back to as well as she was before. Recently she has gone into congested heart failure and needs a transplant. Her mum says that one of Lorraine's biggest fears is that she wont 'love' people in the same way, because she wont have her heart. She's terrified of not being herself when she wakes up. Bless her. Then I left as she came back from theatre, but I will go back tomorrow to see her.

Dan, one of my oldest and best friends text me yesterday saying that his Dad passed away in the morning. He had cancer and in the end, died at home with Dan, his sister, brother and their mum; all there with him, by his side. He had been deteriorating steadily over the last month and it must have been so hard for them to see their dad become iller and iller, weaker and weaker.

Today Dan called me and I spoke to him for 50 minutes. So pleased I did and that he wanted and could talk to me. He said that at the funeral they do not want any flowers. They want all donations to be sent to Great Ormond Street Hospital – because of me. I was so, so moved when Dan said that. So deeply moved. Dan said he'd been keeping his dad – Steve – up to date with my transplant and recovery and biopsies and that his dad was so pleased to know what's been happening up here. I've known Dan and his family for about 22years, so am really close to them. Also Tom is really good friends with Dan's older brother, Chris.

Well for the rest of the day I started typing up my journal with this voice recognition software I bought, which is really good. John made a lovely Ham and Egg Salad for dinner which was really nice. We've all been getting on so well. They just adore Alex!!

Oh, got a parcel from my mate Vale; lovely card and a brand new England top in preparation for the World Cup. Am so touched. They are so expensive and for him to buy it for me by himself is just so nice. I really appreciated it and it fits like a dream.

You should see me, the new 'Supercharged Max' (a phrase me and Pam have been using) with my football top and long hair back with my hair band, like a David Beckham, or Massimo Ambrosini. I well look the part – at least I think so … or just perhaps hope so. The jury is probably still out!

Ever since I have been growing my hair from a No.2 over the past year and a half, my target 'look' or haircut has changed from Fernando Torres, to Heath Ledger in 'A Knights Tale', to James May from 'Top Gear'. But I've now settled on Marlon Brando in 'Mutiny on the Bounty'. Excellent. I look the spit of him – I tell you. Well, hair wise anyway.

Day 34 – 05/06/10

We all went to the seaside today! Cullercoats Beach, Tynemouth. Only 15 minutes drive away. Was wonderful.

WEEK 11

Day 36 – 07/06/10

Okay, haven't written much lately. I think all being well that I should be able to go home next week maybe and therefore have decided to bring this Transplant Journal to an end the day I arrive back at my house. I will write about coming home and in some respects, the end of the 'having a transplant' journey. But like everything, when the pages stop being inked and I put this pen down, that, by no means spells the end of transplantation. I will have rejection episodes and other scares, I'm sure, down the line. But as far as actually being transplanted goes and closing the door on my old life and opening a door to a new one, well that story – this journal – will be brought to a close then; when I open my front door and walk through…

Had such a lovely time with John and Jen. They spoil Alex rotten – it's so wonderful to see. They're always playing with him, walking around with him holding his hands, talking and joking with him.

The beach was lovely. Then we had lunch at Dean and Daniella's and then chilled at home and had a lovely roast-pork, salad dinner. Since they've been here we've played Nomi most nights and I just haven't laughed so much since transplant. They are such wonderful company.

John and Jen left yesterday and I spent the morning dictating my journal to the computer. Then I went on such a mad walk with Alex. Was about 3-4 miles I reckon, all the way down to the railway bridge, along the river and over – took a wrong track and ended up walking three quarters of the way up the ravine on the Jesmond side, then came down, crossed back over the river and walked back up the ravine on another unknown track and ended up by the width restriction way over past the hospital and down the road. So followed the road to the David Lloyd Gym, round the whole Paddy Freeman's Park and home (with a cheeky strawberry ice-cream by the lake) in about an hour and fifteen minutes? Say about 4 miles. I ascended that ravine twice pushing Alex and I didn't stop once – and was walking at a decent speed.

At the top of the second main ascent I felt my heart beating faster than it has, as of yet. But the faster it beats, the more power I feel, the more strength I feel tear through my body, the more life I feel course through my cardio-vascular system. It's just a constant, constant high. I am on Cloud 9. I am in my Nirvana.

But... but today... for some reason especially today, that feeling, that plateau that my life has ascended to, right now makes it so, so hard for me. Because of home. Because of my family back home, my brother and the polar-opposite world they are in.

I will keep this brief as what I am going to write, in light of Tom and Liza and my family's grief at the loss of Baby Jack, is so, so selfish. I wasn't going to write it, but I will. I have never felt so apart, so estranged, so distant from my family. Me, Mum, Tom, Emma and Louise are all so close. And yet, I have never been so in a different world, so further away from them ever. Even when me and Pam were staying in Methern, New Zealand – probably as far away as I could get from home, did I ever feel this lonely.

And it's so simple to explain. I'm on that plateau, and the rest of my family are gripped in grief. I cannot, as much as I've tried, get anywhere near their pain, because I can't be there. And to some extent, they cannot see the view from this plateau I'm living on, which day by day is greater and more spectacular, whilst they descend further and further into the core of their tragedy. They are crying and dreading the funeral – seeing a 2ft coffin disappear behind the curtain to be committed to ash – and I am buzzing from my walk and discovering highs I didn't even know existed. They are writing poems and thoughts to go into little Jack's 'Order of Service' book and I am planning what I can aspire to do next and how wonderful it is. In short, I can't wait for tomorrow and the others, especially Tom and Liza, probably can't even care for tomorrow. And therein lies the intraversable distance and irreconcilable difference between us.

I have never been so alone or estranged from my family. And it is unbearable. Truly unbearable. It, I get the sense, is extremely hard for Mum too, because she, unlike the others (I think), knows most of my world up here and has been at the sharpest end of the grief back home with Tom and Liza. So she, being the Mum and sole parent of this family, is being torn both ways. I am worried the opposing fortunes and stages of her children's lives and the opposing force that this inflicts on her, may well pick her apart. Because of the strength of the opposing forces and conflict that ultimately this will create in her, as she is only one person and can only be in one place at a time.

She said in a letter to me that she is struggling with an impossible situation – she wouldn't elucidate, but she didn't need to. I mean, I'm not even allowed to the funeral which, I now think, is a bad idea. I should be there. I'm Tom's brother. But it's not my decision and I will never be bitter about it – just sad.

So you can see why Mum is being pulled apart by such opposing needs in her two sons, knowing she can't satisfy both as much as she wants. She also put in her letter that she cannot wait for our family to be reunited. Boy, neither can I. Not sure how much of this loneliness and estrangement I can take. Am already taking it out badly on Pam which I must stop – sorry Pam. Not too long now hopefully, hopefully, hopefully. Just to go with all this I wanted to stick in a photo of Jack and Tom which mum sent in her letter. I love you both, you two – father and son. Love you xxx

Original Journal contained a picture of baby Jack laying, in just his little nappy, on Tom's bare-chest – both with their eyes closed, in those last minutes together.

This is the most painfully beautiful picture I have ever seen.

I have always struggled to understand the line in that wonderful poem by an Indian elder called, 'Oria Mountain Dreamer.' The line is:

'I want to know if you can see beauty, even when it's not pretty'.

Looking at that photo of Tom and Jack, I now understand.

Day 38 – 09/06/10

John is coming back up today to help us out. He's been such a source of help and support for us. We are going into Newcastle to meet him at about 11 AM. We'll try to get some nice lunch out I reckon, although the weather is overcast and drizzly so probably wont want to wander around too much.

Had outpatient review yesterday. 7:30-11 AM as always – such a long morning. Gareth isn't in this week so saw one of the Adult-team Surgeons instead – apparently he was the one who took out my ICD. He was nice. Said I'm doing really well and everything is looking good except my blood-pressure, which is still higher than they would like, but no major problem – just something they'll keep their eye on.

Really, all being well at my next outpatient review and biopsy on the 15th, I should be allowed to go home. Man what a moment that will be! Still, don't want to get too excited. I haven't got my blood test results yet from yesterday so until I get those I'll keep a lid on my excitement.

Had another real long, hilly walk with Alex yesterday. Was out for about two hours. Walked over to Jesmond, had a foot-long subway and then looped back to the lake and had the nicest ice-cream ever; rhubarb and vanilla, mmmn...

My mate Eddy is coming to visit tomorrow. Arriving tomorrow night and leaving Saturday morning, so get a whole day with him. Am so pleased and looking forward to it. Haven't seen my friends since coming up here. And it's so nice of Eddy to come up just by himself and not to wait for anyone else. I really admire and think a lot of him for that.

Anyway as this whole place now, even when I'm over the hospital, feels like the 'wind down' to going home, I'll probably write very little from now on – unless something significant happens of course, because everything, as I wrote a few days ago, feels sort of like this is all coming to an end.

I'll keep you updated as best I can, however the time to move on is coming I feel. I have started to become more reminiscent when sitting at this Journal's pages, rather than wanting to just write about what's happening. I suppose that signifies a coming of a change. But I don't want to tempt fate any further. Just wanted to explain that so you don't get disgruntled, or feel ignored if I do not write in you for days on end. It's not because I've forgotten about you. Far from it. It's because that maybe I do not need you in the same way now. And that feat is to both our credits.

Am I actually writing to my Journal? I've been up here too long! I must be going mad, writing to a bundle of paper, bound in a cheap faux suede sleeve. But, as I'm sure you're aware, anytime I address my Journal, I am really just talking to myself or that part of myself, which has stood inside me, observing and listening, and always seeing me for who I really am – without any pre, or miss-conceptions. The perfect yard stick. The purest listening post; my conscience – plain and simple. I'll say bye for now. May well be a short while before I write in you again, maybe not.... so many things we can never ever know.

Day 41 – 12/06/10

Told you it could be a while before I wrote in you again! Well a good few things have happened I suppose. On Wednesday I called up for my blood test results and all meds remained unchanged, but the main piece of news – which I was so pleased about – was that I no longer needed a midweek blood test between check-ups (usually on a Friday). So for the first time since I've been up here, I've got nothing that needs checking or testing for a whole week! Tuesday to Tuesday, that's what awaits me. And what made me so happy is that now I've been pushed out to weekly checks, unless something bad happens – rejection or infection – then I'm sure I'll be allowed to go home next week. Again though I still don't want to tempt fate – but it's looking good.

Eddy come up Thursday night. His flight was delayed so he didn't get here until 10:30 PM, but was such a good visit. We both sat up until midnight chatting with a few cervezas which was really nice. I read him 'The Waterfall Ascent' – that's what I'm calling my Journal entry under 20/05/10. It looked like it really moved him.

Then had a lovely full day with him on the Friday. Something I'm ashamed, or even a little embarrassed to write, considering that Friday was little Jack's funeral. But I'll tell you briefly, only briefly however, what that was like – through the voice of Emma, sister-Lou and Mum, who told me about it over the phone, later.

At 10:20 AM me and Eddy went into the Chapel, as that was

the scheduled time of Jack's funeral service. We sat, not in silence, just casually and talked about a few things, but mainly Jack, Tom, Liza and Mum. Told Eddy a lot about it and then, near the end, I played Tom's song, 'I'm Wondering Why?' The nice Chaplain, who I've talked to the most – Kathy – came in and asked me how I was and if I needed anything – especially someone to talk to, as she will always be there … so nice.

Then me and Eddy just had such a nice day. Walked into Newcastle as the weather changed from mild and cloud covered, to warm with blue skies and blazing sunshine. We walked all the way down to the Quayside.

Had a few beers in a few pubs at the Quayside – bumped into cousin Dan who was there on a stag-do along with 24 others! Then walked back up to town to watch the first game in the FIFA World Cup 2010 – South Africa (the hosts) versus Mexico. We watched it at Lineker's Bar; 3 PM kick-off so the bar wasn't very busy, which I was thinking about, considering my immuno-suppression. However, due to the dreariness of the first half's football, 0-0, we left the bar and had a nice walk back.

On route me and Eddy put on an accumulator bet at Ladbrooks – all the group winners except for Group A which had already kicked off. Me, Eddy and Tom each put in £10 (Eddy put in for Tom). No idea what we'd win – haven't got a clue how to work it out! We got back at about 5 PM so was out all day; legs were well aching. We must of clocked up the miles.

Then that evening me and Eddy got a blow out Chinese takeaway and watched the second game, France V's Uruguay at home with John – Pam unsurprisingly, retired to bed early.

*   *   *

Eddy left at 5:30 AM this morning as he had a 7 AM flight back, so I didn't get to see him off. But was such a treat being with a mate. Felt so normal again, just so very, very normal. He took one and a half days off work, spent over £100 on the flight and travelled up and down all by himself just to see me for a day. So wonderful. Am so very touched.

On the Friday morning Pam had her Thyroid appointment with Pedros Petros, who Pam said was extremely nice and competent. Pam's thyroid Dr in Basildon, Dr Kahn, said that in his opinion Dr Petros was the world's foremost leader in Endocrinology – a heavy accolade.

Dr Petros said that Pam has Graves disease, where her body thinks its thyroid isn't hers and attacks it. Says it's nothing too bad so don't be worried, just need regular blood tests (especially during pregnancy) and will need to take thyroid medicine.

At present her thyroid is now balanced, so during this pregnancy she should be ok. He spent 45 minutes with her explaining all about it, what to look out for and all sorts. And to top that all off Dr Petros gave Pam his personal mobile number and said if she has any problems to call him directly – how nice is that. The healthcare me and Pam have received up here has been absolutely extraordinary!

I suppose I should tell you a bit about the funeral, but only a bit. Mum, Tom and Liza, Em, Lou, Dan, Matt, Sarah, Steve and Liza's friend Natalie, Reverend Ed Morris and little resting baby Jack, filled the Chapel at the Crematorium. Tom, in his arms alone, carried Jack in his beautiful, pure-white, tiny casket into the Chapel and laid him upon the altar.

Three songs played through the still air: 'Mad World', 'Tears in Heaven' and 'The Sound of Silence'. The reason they played those three is because Tom played those songs the most at home on his piano to Jack when he was growing inside his Mum.

Then the Reverend said a few really nice words and then read out a poem written by Tom. I may write in the poem, but I think probably not. I will ask Tom later, much much later. Then the Reverend read a short part out of what Mum wrote, it was a short letter written to Jack which started, 'Sad day today baby...'

Then all of them, except the Reverend and except Jack, went to the country pub near where Tom and Liza live and stayed there for a few hours. And then the funeral was over.

There were so many tears at the funeral. So, so many tears – gut crawling, cork screwing spasms of grief and tortuous straining of trying to 'hold in' louder cries that could have chilled heaven, no doubt.

All of them felt the true power of grief in that Chapel. All of them felt the loss and the wonder of what a funeral actually is: a goodbye; everlasting; enduring; perpetual and final. Goodbyes are always sad and yesterday was perhaps the hardest goodbye anyone could ever have to say. But Mum said the service, although brief, was in its own rights deeply perfect and wonderful. But what Tom wrote I just can't tell you. I hope you get to read it. It's.... it's.... well, I can't tell you. I just can't.

Day 43 – 14/06/10

Will only really tell you about two main things over the last few days. Firstly baby Alex. He has just raced ahead in development and is now oh so close to walking. He did yesterday take – what me and Pam have decided to call – his official, first steps. He's been standing, holding onto us, the settee, his play table and stuff for a while now. And in the last month has wanted to walk around everywhere whilst you walk behind him, leaning over, holding his two, up-stretched hands. He plods along walking from this room to the next taking all his own weight and a fair chunk of balance too, but not enough to be able to let go of our hands.

So a few days ago Pam bought a baby-walker (kind of like a little shopping trolley without the basket/trolley part to it) for Alex to be able to push around and walk – aided, but only by himself. It's a further stage of walking development as, although his balance is still aided, all adjustments to keep balanced and walking he makes himself. There is no intelligent help being given in the form of me, or John holding his hands, using our strength, balance, or knowledge to correct any over tilting or unstable listing.

So using the baby walker, Alex learnt really quickly to walk in straight lines, from one side of the living room to the other; all in one piece. Was wonderful to see. It's quite an achievement as well, because Alex has to adjust and adapt his walking pace in line with the resistance the walker has against the carpet. If he pushes the walker ahead too fast without increasing his walking pace, he would go head first into the floor and if he doesn't go forward with enough strength, the walker wont move and he'll fall backwards, or just remain standing.

But Alex negotiated and navigated his way through these perils with only a few spills, to now be, pretty much, fully proficient at straight-line walking with his baby-walker. But obviously those were not his first steps...

Alex's first steps were yesterday when I was sitting on the floor with him. As always Alex hated being on the floor, so he decided to get onto his feet by climbing up my knee, then onto my arm, then, pushing his bum in the air and straightening up his back, he was standing; just lightly placing one hand on my shoulder for balance.

As he was stable I shimmied back a touch so that he was standing by himself – something he has done before for a good 10-20 seconds. Anyway this time he wasn't satisfied with standing, so he took his first few steps forward to get back to me. However, as he done that, I quickly shimmied back further. When Alex got to where I was before my shimmying he stopped, stood still and smiled very briefly.

Then he walked another few steps to get to where I was, but again I shimmied backwards. Although this only lasted a few seconds and say about 6-8 steps, Alex was walking – there's no doubt about it.

His amble only came to an end because I couldn't shimmy back any further, as I had hit the sofa, therefore Alex finally caught me and flew his arms around my neck with his adorable smile. But he done it. His first few, controlled steps. On the 13th July 2010; marked, stamped and official ... my baby boy has walked! He's learning so fast, he really is. Bless him.

The second thing I'm going to tell you is about today and another 'Eureka' moment; an even greater Eureka moment than 'The Waterfall Ascent' – and just as moving. I will be however, much briefer than the waterfall's description, safe in the knowledge that what I felt on that ascent was the same as today, except that today I was a little higher than before, in my new-life-flight from my aforementioned old-life's marshland of physical struggle, to the furthest reaches of that universe of possibility.

We started at the bottom of the car park at the base of Durham historic city mount. We then walked up the steep hills and old cobbled streets to Durham Cathedral. I pushed Alex up the steep incline to the summit of the hill, where Durham Cathedral and other monastic buildings all stood, atop the whole of county Durham.

Then we went inside the imposing Cathedral and saw that the tower was open for ascent. Me and John paid £5 each and I ignored the warning sign that said anyone with heart problems should not attempt the climb.

We entered a wide, pleasant, spiral staircase at the foot of the north transept. We ascended up the stairs past the pier of tall, stone columns, above the arcade, over the triforium and then, rising atop the clerestory, we came to the base of the tower.

Then the wide, spiral staircase turned into an impossibly narrow, much steeper and more uneven, jagged spiral staircase. It was sort-of the point of no return. A tiny, cramped, claustrophobic ascent to the top of the tower. Only a couple of cut-in doorways were there to rest in.

Other than that it was just up and up and up. Step after step after step. No view except the stone ahead, to my left, to my right, the floor and a few inches above my head. Entombed. Entombed in stone. No view. No point of reference. No idea how many steps left, or how high up you were; other than the odd embrasure letting in a slit of light and a tiny abstraction of the outside world.

All you have is your thoughts. Your perception of your fatigue and the stone ... the suffocating, narrowing stone.

I was nervous, scared and unsure of myself. These are the moments where I really build up trust and faith in my new heart. And after a while we reached the top of the tower and the highest point of Durham county. I couldn't believe it. 325 steps it was – 70 meters. And I went up every step with only one, tiny rest midway. Unbelievable.

I briefly thought of all of those times I've not been able to do what I had just done: The Monument with Mum – had to turn back. St Paul's Cathedral with family – no way could I attempt that ascent. Windsor Castle on a school trip, York Cathedral on family holiday with my Dad's side of the family. Valencia Castle recently when me and Pam were there and probably many more also.

Now I can do them. I can make it. I CAN. Now I simply CAN! I cannot tell you what it feels like.

Atop the tower John walked over to the parapet and looked out around the 360 degree, panoramic view of Durham county and out through the neighbouring counties; Northumberland and Cumbria. The sky wasn't clear, but the clouds were light and so high up that they did not impede the view at all.

John said to come and look at the view as I, once getting to the tower's roof, took a well deserved break and sat on the wooden, apex roof. I thought to myself, I don't need to see it – that's not why I came up here. Whatever the view ... whatever its beauty... whatever its sweeping, distant, clear and remarkable sight... it would undoubtedly be insignificant, drab, vapid

and even insipid compared to the feeling of joy and glory,
already burning like an inferno, deep inside me.

Of course I did get up and look at the view and it was
beautiful. But the achievement was far greater. Once back in
the Nave, I lit a tea-light candle and wrote down the below
prayer;

> # Jack
>
> # Michael
>
> # Andrew
>
> # Steve
>
> # Sleep Peacefully

Today was Steve's – Dan's dad – funeral. It felt really good to
write that prayer. The four deaths I have been touched by since
being here...

Day 46 – 17/06/2010

Today could be, well – to tell you the truth – most likely *will* be, a
momentous day. It's noon and at 1.30 PM I've got to phone the
Transplant Outpatient clinic to get my biopsy results. If all is okay
... I'M GOING HOME!!!!!!!!! Unbelievable. But before I get into
that, let me tell you about a few things over the last few days.

On Tuesday (15th) I was all geared up for going to
Outpatients for my full review and biopsy with the hope that
they would, either let me go home there-and-then, or possibly
the next day. Couldn't sleep the night before. I awoke at 5 AM

and just couldn't drift back off – such was my excitement.

Anyhow, killed some time and went to clinic bright and breezy at 7.30 AM full of anticipation. Mary, one of the Outpatient nurses, came over to me as I was waiting with all of the others and said, 'Max, your biopsy is for the 16th.'

I said I know (I remember writing the date down thinking, oh that's next Tuesday)

Then she said – as the penny just wasn't dropping with me – 'Max, today is the 15th!'

Shucks. Better keep that blooper under my hat. Double shucks – have just written it in the Journal for all who read it to see. Oh nevermind. I did just have a Heart Transplant only 6 weeks ago you know! Wonder how long I can play that card for?

So just bowed my head and left the clinic with an embarrassed air of ignominy. Only joking, they said it's an easy mistake to make.

So, Outpatient review and biopsy take two. This time on the 16th; Wednesday the 16th, not Tuesday the 16th! In the waiting room I saw Alan and Jenny, the Northern-Irish couple I briefly spoke about at the start of Journal 1. Jenny had a double-lung transplant a couple of weeks before we arrived up here and was just attending her 3-weekly check-up. Was lovely to run into them again. Such lovely, lovely people. She looks so well and is back to full health almost, which is amazing considering she was unwell and on oxygen for 3 years previous. We exchanged phone numbers and we both wished each other well.

Then in the biopsy recovery room I got talking to this woman who was also having a biopsy. I've spoken to her before at Outpatients previously. She's late 40's and had her heart transplant 13 weeks ago. However, talking to her about rejection made me realise why I've found it so easy and un-unnerving having someone else's heart inside me...

When she was transplanted her heart immediately started to reject. So much so that the heart went into quite severe distress and they couldn't even close her chest for a good few hours.

Then a week later, her heart started to reject again. Apparently there are two types of rejection: when your body rejects the heart and, much rarer and harder to treat, when the heart itself actually rejects the body. And it was this much rarer rejection that this woman – didn't catch her name – had.

The rejection needed to be strongly treated with complicated plasma transfers, which eventually brought it under control. However, during the rejection episode, when the heart was not working properly, she really swelled – also due to the meds too. The swelling became so severe around her chest that her wound actually burst open! She had to go back down to Theatre for 3 hours for re-stitching and clamping. And when she returned her neat, straight, sternum scar looked like zig-zag slashes; like she'd been mauled.

The reason I'm telling you all of this, is because of one very simple, very easy-to-understand concept. The woman has, even after 13 weeks, very little confidence, or trust in her new heart, because she thinks that the heart itself doesn't want to be there.

She said that it instantly started to reject – the heart rejected her – not the other way around. And rejected her so much her chest burst open, like it was trying to escape. Since then, although she is now very well, she still cannot walk up a hill by herself. She can with others, but does not have the confidence to do it alone with her new heart.

You see in her mind her and her new heart are both separate entities and she feels that her heart doesn't want to be there. So she is really struggling with the knowledge of, not so much having someone else's heart, but thinking that her heart is not on her side, or not part of her team. And conversely this is why I've found it so easy to accept and live with my new heart, because at transplant the heart was extremely strong – supercharged – and when transplanted it instantly started contracting extremely well, with excellent systolic function and it also went straight into sinus rhythm. Straight away it was happy; content; willing … ready to pump away, powerfully and peacefully. And since then I have not had, as yet, any rejection.

So you see, instantly, as soon as I regained consciousness and evermore-so with each day that I achieve more and more, I have become a team with Andrew's heart. We are, although still separate in origin, together and 'at one' with each other in much more than just physical, literal terms.

That's why, I realise now, I've found the concept of having someone else's heart in me so untroublesome – because it straight away became a part of 'Team Max.' Like my prosthetic tricuspid valve and I.C.D before it, it is now at home, at peace and 'singing from the same song sheet' as me. I know some people say that it is my heart now, but to me it will always be Andrew's heart. But Andrew's heart that is now working for me and seemingly happy to be doing so too.

Happy heart, happy mind! Thanks Andrew, I owe you.

Well that's taken me to 12.52 PM. 38 minutes until I find out if I can go home!!!!!

EEEEEK! Am so excited and nervous. But those emotions are pretty much synonymous a lot of the time. I hope I can go home. Hopefully. Hopefully. Hopefully. . .

As I wrote in an email to Pat: *Home is an inner peace that can no further be added to by the addition of anything you can think of . . .* And: *Home is where the heart is. . .*

35 minutes and counting . . . EEEEK. . . ..

The following text not in original Journal but added later by me:

Biopsy was clear therefore all four of us drove straight home in our tiny Fiesta on the 17th. That night we – except John – stayed round Mum's as we had no cot at home. The next morning my family, Me, Pam, Alex and bump (along with Mum's cot we borrowed until we move our stuff back from Newcastle) drove the short 10 minutes from Mum's to our house; HOME. We stayed in all day and I just took it all in; bit-by-bit. After our first night back in our bed and our first morning all together in our family home, I knew it was time to conclude the Journal.

End of post-Journal Insert

Day 48 – 19/06/10 – Final Transplant Journal Entry

'Wow. What a ride...'
I made it back.
I made it home
I made it.

79 nights, 78 days, family relocation, a rented house, one heart transplant, four deaths, one fated birth, one promise of a new life, one wedding, two funerals, Graves disease, triumph and tragedy – heart loss, heart gain and heart break.
So much. Oh so much.
All the fear and uncertainty, doubt and worry, hope and possibility, prayer and wish, faith and love...
I have endured so much: loneliness and weariness, physical pain and discomfort, The Valley of the Shadow of Death and the realisation of a dream...
I have faced possibly the greatest crossroad a man can face: one path death and the other my most wild and impossible dreams. Annihilation, or the ability to fly. Utter despair and unbearable suffering for my wife and baby-son, or a new, stronger, faster, fitter, healthier, abler, better husband and father to keep. It is the most heady prospect to consider – the void between success and failure could not have been any greater.
I've never felt more connected and loved by my family and yet, at times, distant and estranged from them.
I've never felt more complete than when I awoke this

morning, in my bed, in my home, with my wife and my son –
but I've never felt so at a loss as to how to appreciate and move
on from these last 78 days.

I've never known joy, or bliss, or spirit like what I have felt
through these Journals.

I've never known fear, or distance, or longing, or loneliness
than what I have experienced through these Journals.

But I am Home. Home. Home.

It's my same lovely home, near my wonderful family, by my
close friends – the epicentre of my whole life. And although
these are all the same, just as I left them, everything I remembered and expected them to be, they are all, now, sitting under
a different sky, under different stars - for I am much changed.
And my world will be so different from now on.

And I suppose this is the penultimate thought I want to end
on. I have done it. I made it. Although I'm still only 6 weeks out
from transplant and the real safe barriers come at 3 months and
then 1 year, and therefore the transplant journey is far from
over – indeed will never really be over. But now I'm home and
well and have made it back, I am ready, now ready, to start my
new life. What dreams may come…

I said 'penultimate' because the last words in these Journals
have to be a dedication; an overriding and enduring honouring
of one person. Plenty of people are due my thanks and
gratitude. Certain members of my family are due my never-
ending and everlasting love and most deepest respect; Mum
and John especially. Two people mainly I owe my life to; Andrew
and Dr Asif Hasan.

But, most of all, more than any other this Journal, with all its
words and all my life I dedicate and give, unreservedly to my
wife: Pamela Tricia Crompton. To you Pam, I owe it all. Thanks
Honey. I Love you…

Well goodbye my Journal and God Bless. Thanks for your
company.

'See you later…'

Other Writings

Letter to Alex as I was rushed for transplant in December.

Written: 18th December 2009 @ 21:20

Alex, have just got a call for a possible heart transplant and I wanted to write to you just in case things don't turn out too well.

I should have written this sooner whilst I was waiting on the list, however I'm dreadfully unorganised!! Am sorry :-)

I love you so much Alex. That's the first and main thing I need to say. You and your Mum are the best things that have ever happened to me and my time with you both has been the happiest and fullest of my life.

I want you to live the best life you know how to, and also always listen to Mummy, because she knows best.

I won't give you much advice, because I trust you and I trust your upbringing by your mother, to already have all the sound advice you would need.

But I will just say to be a 'giver' as much as you can, not a 'taker' – your uncle Tom will explain.

You are so gorgeous my son, from the day you were born to now. I can't tell you how perfect you are.

I will again leave it up to your Mum, your Nan and aunts and uncles to tell you about me and who I am – I hope you like the vicarious version :-) !

I could carry on writing for days, but I've got to go.

I love you so much my son.

Daddy

xxx

Letter to my Donor family:

Written: 14th July 2010

To Andrew's Family – my heart donor.

It has taken me fifteen minutes to even decide how to address this letter; this letter which is the hardest that I have ever written. And in light of such difficulty I will start with the opening line from a letter my family received from the Transplant Office when we, jointly, decided to donate my father's liver, a few years ago now: 'I hope that time is treating you gently in these early weeks after Andrew's loss . . .'

You see comfort and peace are foreign lands, it seems, when someone so loved and dear is taken from us. But I know that – despite the void of gratitude and debt that I owe to Andrew and yourselves, which I will never be able to fill – that writing to you to tell you something of me and my journey may, just may, offer a glimpse of comfort, or a shimmer of peace. In such painful and turbulent seas this is a tall task, I know, but one which I must try my hardest to do.

Andrew has done much, much more than just save my life. That's for sure. I was born with a congenital heart condition and although I have lived a mostly normal life – up until recently when I became critically unwell – I have never been able to exert myself physically, as my heart just never had the strength ... I could not play football with my friends, go on long walks that involved hills, play any sports really, go bike riding, walk up three or four flights of stairs, run, skip, play tag, or rounders in Primary School. And a whole host more.

The reason I am telling you this is that now, with Andrew's gift, with Andrew's wonderfully strong heart, I have started, even in these early months after surgery, doing things that I have never been able to do. Again, I could tell you many things that I have done in the last month, which I never could have dreamed of doing before, however I'll mention just one: when I was discharged from hospital after the transplant, one of the first things I done was to go and buy a push bike. Then I went on a 17 mile bike ride with my Mum; I have never been able, in my life, to go bike riding with Mum. When cycling along we both had tears in our eyes.

And this is what I want to say overridingly and emphatically; that Andrew did not just save my life, he has not just given me many more years here to see my young family grow, he has – on top of all of that – given me a new life – a new quality of life – which is literally making my most wild and impossible dreams come true. For so many years I have had to miss out on so many things, but now I can take part; I can keep up, I can live a fuller and richer life than me, or any of my family, ever thought possible. I have always compared the idea of me being able to run, to a normal person being able to fly. Well, a few weeks ago, I ran on a treadmill for the first time…Andrew has quite literally given me wings.

My wife is currently pregnant with our second child and we have decided that the baby's middle name will be, Andrew if it's a boy and Andie if it's a girl. As soon as we found out that she was pregnant I knew, within that instant, that that is was I wanted to do. I owe Andrew and you everything – absolutely everything – and this is just one tiny, tiny thing that I can do to honour and remember Andrew and his unspeakably generous gift.

Well I have no idea, as maybe you do not either, as to whether, or not, this letter is too long, too detailed, too personal, too painful … but I didn't know how to go about writing such a letter, so I thought the best thing I could do is be myself and write from the heart – so to speak.

I do hope I have not offended you in anyway and that this letter – at least some of it – will show you the unsurpassable goodness and unquantifiable joy and happiness that has been borne out of such generosity and tragedy. Again, I do hope that you can find at least a little peace, at least a little rest from the pain by knowing what has become of Andrew's heart . . .

Thank-you all so very, very much.

Max, 27 years old.

My Thank-you letter to the Freeman Hospital
Written: Monday, 02 August 2010

To: Asif, Massimo, Amanda, Debbie, John, Milind, David, Lynne, Kirsty, Neil and all related teams

Well. What can I say. I knew I wanted to write a thank-you letter to the team, but now it comes to it, I'm temporarily out of words...

Let me tell you what I've been thinking about. I have been feeling kind of sorry for you all, in a funny way. Let me explain.

The job you all do must be very rewarding, amongst many other things, I'm sure. But I imagine – and I may be wrong – that when you all, as a team, raise someone away from pain and suffering and return them to happiness . . . return them to being pink . . . return them to living life, in all its bittersweet splendour, you must feel so good. You must be really pleased and proud of yourselves and the team as a whole.

However, I know (I think) that none of you have a congenital heart disease. None of you have ever lived with the effects of chronic heart failure. None of you have had to stand there, on the side-line, with the teacher, whilst all the other kids are sprinting around – free – playing football at will and at ease...

I am coming to my point soon; honestly! You see what I'm trying to say, is no matter how much you see of it in your work, for no matter how long, or for how many hours a day . . . a week . . . a year . . . a career – you cannot know, implicitly, of the pain or struggle of living with a congenital heart disease.

And therefore – and this is my point – you cannot at all appreciate the joy, the heavenly bliss of being saved from such diseases and such limitations. You can't know the good you do. You can't know the wonderful impact and effect you have on peoples lives and their families. You cannot appreciate your own work, because you cannot know, really know, of the happiness you bring to people.

And, in a roundabout way, this is why I have felt strangely sorry for you. Because you are creating such joy in this world, you are creating such happiness, you are giving oh so, so much goodness back into this world and you do not know – can not know – of it all. And it's such a shame because you so deserve to know and understand and appreciate the good you do. You really all do. But no matter what, you just can't.

It must really be something you know, helping people the way you do. But I just want you to know that whatever pride, or satisfaction, or warmth, or joy you feel from helping people like me, just remember, that however much of those feelings you feel, they should be multiplied by near on infinity before you get anywhere close to justly reaping the rewards of your work.

Ultimately, I suppose, you will never be rewarded enough for the work you do. And perhaps the gap between what you all as a team deserve and the joy you feel at making someone better, is a gap that can be filled by the knowledge of how highly you are all thought of; by me, my family, my friends and I'm sure many, many more of your other patients.

I have never been to a hospital like The Freeman. I have never been part of a medical care team such as the Paediatric and Transplant Team at The Freeman. It is something extremely special . . . much more than any other hospital I have been to. I don't know why and I don't know if I can really put my finger on it – it just feels like . . . like . . . home. If that makes any sense at all?

Well, I am conscious of rambling and taking up too much of your precious time . . . golden time – that's what I think I'll call the time you spend at work. Apparently they called Dr Barnard 'the man with the golden hands.' Well, I think I'll plagiarise and call you all, collectively, 'the team with the golden touch'

Along with my donor, you have all changed my life so much. I'll never be able to tell you how much, or thank you enough. And that's something we will both have to live with – however, please know that you have done more for me and my family than anyone could ever do for someone. Collectively there is nothing greater, within humanity's bravest sword, that anyone could ever do, than that of which you have done for me.

True greatness is hard to come by. But it's everywhere you look at The Freeman

God bless to you all and all of your families . . .

Thank-you with all of my old and new heart

Max

Intensive Care Anniversary (Written one year on from my Cardiac Arrest)

Written: 20/09/2009 @ 19.50

This exact time last year I was in Intensive care. My wife was rubbing my fluid loaded feet, whilst my mum held both my hands. I was breathing through an oxygen mask with the spray of the gas misting my glasses from clear to fogged and back again with every breath. Every breath, which had, in the recent waking hours, taken on such new meaning.

The constant clouding of my glasses impaired my vision, but my view of the world was far more distorted by the news that I was given, only hours before. I couldn't believe it. I scarcely dared to. I had travelled down the road to death, but seemed to have been brought back at the last crossroad.

I was just staring out, at Pam, and at mum, both of them coming into and falling out of focus with each mist, of each breath, and I could not take in the world that laid out in front of me. I was in shock, no doubt. My body the day before had been subjected to life threatening trauma and I was feeling the effects on every level. I was, as far as my consciousness goes, at rock bottom. Shattered and pounded. Pounded by wave upon wave of torturous discovery and that sense of utter disbelief. Just relentless pounding resonating, it seems, with the rhythm of each breath upon my glasses; in and out, cloudy and clear, disbelief and despair.

*   *   *

That was last year. Now things are much changed. This morning I laid lazily in bed, on this Sunday morning with Pam and with our three-week-old, to-the-day, baby boy, Alex James. I was precariously propped up against the bedstead with only one pillow – Pam had all the others giving her a much more comfortable posture. She says she needs them for breast feeding support, but I'm not sure if I buy that. Especially when beautiful baby Alex, at the precise time, was laying snugly along my thighs with our cover laying gently over him.

I had kinked my knees so he was laying at an angle facing me and Pam with the window behind, pouring soft autumnal morning light, warmly over his adorable face. He was as contented as could be – his inescapably large, navy blue eyes, were darting back and fourth, up and down and with every new stare his little lips and ever podgier cheeks, moved through expression after expression, with a carefree abandon and randomness only possible with newborns.

Us three laid there for some time. I put our music on. And we just laid there, me and Pam, both starring at Alex with an intensity that he was, no doubt, looking out with also. The morning sun stayed constant and our brand new family were enjoying the empty minutes that were falling by without comment or purpose.

Alex yawned. He pursed his lips and tried to look almost behind himself. Pam shifted down her many pillows and tucked her head on my left shoulder, resting on the exact spot which would not push down on my ICD. I slid my little figure between Alex's left hand and he instinctively gripped. Alex's expressions continued, Pam's cuddle remained, and I was looking out at them both and myself, with a similar sense of utter disbelief – except today it was disbelief that one year on, this moment, could be, this perfect.

I wonder, if there could be, at all, a starker contrast between today and this day last year? I dare not to even dread or dream, of this day next year.

Written: 20/09/2010 @ 15.10 (The next 20th September anniversary)

Exactly one year on, to-the-day, from that morning and I am again sitting here, with that same sense of utter disbelief.

In this last year so much has changed. I am a different person, with a different life. What has happened in this past year I can hardly believe. I still scarcely dare too.

How can I sit here today and re-read the last two anniversaries of this date and not tremble? How can I sit here and not feel completely overcome – overrun with what has happened? How can I now 'be', in anyway that I ever knew of 'being'?

Today I sit here, breathing in the air around me, looking out at the courtyard I'm sitting in and I just do not know what to say ... what to write ... or how to describe it.

I suppose all I can say is that last year, I should have dared to 'dream', but even if I had, and even if I'd have dreamt of the most far-reaching, most wildest, most impossible of dreams, I would have fallen far, far short of where I am today; of my life right now, sitting on this bench, with Alex thriving, a little girl on the way and my brand new heart, which has made me physically whole for the first in my life, beating reassuringly inside me.

I wondered last year if there could have been a starker contrast between the two previous anniversaries. Well I've found out that there could be; today. It's today. Except that today it is utter disbelief that another year on, this LIFE, this new life I've been gifted, could be, this perfect.

I will not 'dare' to think about this day next year, because now I just do not need to.

Lightning Source UK Ltd.
Milton Keynes UK

176302UK00007B/10/P